HANGER MANAGEMENT

Also by Susan Albers, PsyD

50 Ways to Soothe Yourself Without Food

50 More Ways to Soothe Yourself Without Food

Eat Q

But I Deserve This Chocolate!

Mindful Eating 101

Eating Mindfully

Eat, Drink & Be Mindful

Eating Mindfully for Teens

HANGER MANAGEMENT

MASTER YOUR HUNGER AND IMPROVE
YOUR MOOD, MIND, AND RELATIONSHIPS

SUSAN ALBERS, PsyD

Little, Brown Spark
New York Boston London

Little, Brown Spark
Hachette Book Group
1290 Avenue of the Americas, New York, NY 10104
littlebrownspark.com

First Edition: December 2019

Little Brown Spark is an imprint of Little, Brown and Company, a division of Hachette Book Group, Inc. The Little, Brown Spark name and logo are trademarks of Hachette Book Group, Inc.

The publisher is not responsible for websites (or their content) that are not owned by the publisher.

The Hachette Speakers Bureau provides a wide range of authors for speaking events. To find out more, go to hachettespeakersbureau.com or call (866) 376-6591.

Hanger Management™ is a registered trademark owned by Susan Albers LLC.

Illustrations by Erwand

ISBN 978-0-316-52456-8
LCCN 2019946443

10 9 8 7 6 5 4 3 2 1

LSC-C

Printed in the United States of America

Contents

Contents

Contents

Preface

The inspiration for this book began eleven years ago—in church.

No, it wasn't divine intervention. It was a moment of sheer embarrassment.

That day in church I had made a grave mistake, but I didn't know it until about twenty minutes into the service.

I remember it vividly. At first, everything was going well. It was like any other Sunday. My eighteen-month-old daughter was smiling and waving, entertaining the people seated around us. I was so proud of her. She looked cute as a button and angelic in a pink, ruffly dress with a pink bow secured in her blond hair.

But then she began to get fussy and wiggly.

I recognized this change in her demeanor immediately and knew exactly what it meant. I smiled and reached calmly into my oversized bag for her Cheerios. My hand fished around the bottom of the bag. Then I began to frantically search the pockets.

Oh no. Did I forget the Cheerios? I thought. These were essential to getting through an hour-long service. *I made the baggie, I know I did.* But then a memory flashed before my eyes: the bag of Cheerios, still sitting on our marble kitchen countertop.

I tried to distract her with her plush Elmo and silly faces, but before my horrified eyes, she began to unravel. She stomped her feet and insisted on her Cheerios. I tried some frantic shushing. The people around me were beginning to give me "that look."

Then, before I knew it, she dashed up the aisle, threw herself down in front of the congregation and had a full-on meltdown. Oh yes. Screaming. Wailing.

I wanted to disappear into the floor. Instead, I dashed to the front to carry her off—arms and feet flailing. As I rushed her out, in front of everyone, my face was a dark shade of crimson.

I had just had an unforgettable lesson in the power of hunger to change our moods.

Let's fast-forward to today. My daughter is a teenager now, but despite all the ways in which she's grown up since that day in church, I still see how the power of food influences her mood.

When I pick her up from school, I can read the emotional climate as soon as the car door shuts. It ranges from "Hey Mom, ask me all about my day!" to "Don't talk to me until I feel human again." True, lots of things besides hunger affect a teenager's mood. But I am still in awe of how big a factor hunger is on that list. So I've learned to wait until we are home and she has had a healthy snack before I ask too many questions about her day. It's worth the wait to hear about what is happening when she has a well-nourished stomach. It's often the difference between a curt "My day was fine" or "Let me tell you all about what happened today, Mom...."

I often talk with my daughter and son about the food and mood connection. Cognitively, they get it. Good food = good mood. Pretty straightforward.

But it wasn't until I took a trip to New York City with my daughter that this concept really hit home for her. My mother, my daughter, and I drove to New York City from Ohio—about eight hours. We started the day with a solid breakfast and had almost reached New Jersey before everyone in the car really began to talk about how hungry they were getting.

I had packed some snacks. My daughter suggested we dig into them so we could skip the mediocre roadside options and focus on finding amazing food in NYC.

I liked this plan. I was dreaming about Thai food in Chelsea.

But to my surprise, my mom crossed her arms and snipped angrily, "I don't want junk. I want food. *Real* food."

My daughter and I exchanged glances. But as my mom had insisted, I drove until I found the next exit.

At the restaurant where we stopped, when my mom went to the bathroom, my daughter tapped me on the shoulder. "I'm sorry for all the things I've ever said when I was hangry," she said earnestly. I knew this word—the combination of *hungry* and *angry*. It was the perfect description of what was happening here.

I smiled internally at my daughter's dead-serious expression. Until that day, she had not witnessed the power of hunger to turn her sweet, mild-mannered grandma into a hungry bear!

"We could all use some hanger management in our lives," I told her. And *voila!* The title for this book was born.

I want to take a moment here for an important caveat. There are many people in the world today who are hungry because they do not have access to food. They are hungry, and sometimes literally starving, for reasons other than the ones that we cover in this book. I don't mention this to provoke guilt. But I think it is important to acknowledge that the hunger I'll be talking about in these pages isn't the type that comes from lack of access to food. It comes from a different problem, and one that we can be grateful for even as we manage it: the struggles we face because we have an abundance of food. Kind of like the way a flood presents a problem different from those caused by a drought.

My hope is that my daughter and son both learn the art of managing their emotional and physical hunger well, so that they can be at their best as young adults—and as adults. And I work in my office at the Cleveland Clinic and through the virtual office of my website (eatingmindfully.com) every day with people who are trying to be their best selves—as parents, employees, students, friends, family members, and significant others.

When we are running on empty—attempting to diet and live on as little food as possible—we are distracted constantly by thoughts of food. Or when we are just plain too busy to make eating well a priority, hunger-induced moodiness can take over. Often, we chalk our bad moods up to stress. In fact, it's the impact of being undernourished—or filled with foods that completely wreck our mood.

But it doesn't have to be that way.

In this book, you will learn about how food can help you to be your best self, too.

Right now, I am smiling. I'm excited to share what I have learned about the psychological power of food.

Thank you for joining me, my kids, and my clients on this journey, turning any hangriness you might have in your life into happiness.

HANGER MANAGEMENT

han•gry

adjective

Bad-tempered or irritable as a result of hunger. A blend of *hungry* and *angry*.

Introduction

"My boyfriend and I almost broke up today. We had been waiting for an hour to be seated at our favorite restaurant. The hostess barely acknowledged our presence. I tapped my foot impatiently. As each moment ticked by, I became more and more hangry. I kept needling him about whether he had gone grocery shopping today. Then I critiqued the list of things he bought. We've been trying to eat healthier. The result? No food in the house. He told me to be quiet and turned away from me. He didn't feel like talking. He said, "I'm starving, what's the freaking holdup?" Eventually, he walked out the door. He stood outside and paced. I screamed out the door for him to just leave. It got ugly, fast. When we are hangry, neither one of us is a rational human being."

—Ava

We've all been there.

All of us have snapped at someone just because we were hungry. And probably someone we know and love has crabbed at us simply because they had a seriously empty belly. When we're not well fed, none of us are at our best. Irritable. Snappy. Downright angry. With my clients, I call this feeling "hangry," a popular term that combines *hungry* and *angry*.

But it's not just being hungry that can ruin our mood. Overeating leads to feelings that are just as unpleasant. Hanger can lead us to overeat, which leaves us feeling what I call "regretfull"—

a combination of *regret* and *full*. It is the physical and emotional discomfort that comes from overeating in a mindless way. I'll explain these concepts in more detail throughout the book. But my guess is that if you are reading this right now, you've experienced them firsthand already. At one time or another, we have all experienced the downright unpleasant feelings that come from being too hungry or overly full.

In my work with thousands of clients in my office and through my virtual practice, I've learned an important truth. Emotions have a huge impact on the way you eat. And what you eat has a significant impact on how you feel. But managing your hunger isn't easy. It's tricky to stay on top of hunger—feeding your stomach just the right amount, not too much and not too little.

The good news is that there are simple, effective strategies for managing hunger-induced moodiness. And strategies that don't just prevent moodiness, but actually boost your mood through eating. Yes, that's right. Eating well can make you feel amazing!

I call it Hanger Management. In this book, we'll get to the bottom of what causes hanger—and how to prevent it. And using the techniques of mindful eating, you'll learn to be on top of your eating habits and at your best. As a special bonus for buying this book, please visit my website, eatingmindfully.com, for freebies to help you kick hanger to the curb.

HANGER MANAGEMENT: IT'S PROBABLY NOT WHAT YOU THINK — AND THAT'S GOOD NEWS!

The other day I went to a birthday party for a colleague of mine who was turning forty. Her husband had it catered, and the dining room table was a sea of desserts, including cookies, cakes, and pie: everything a sweet tooth could desire. As I was standing by the table, eyeing the spread, a woman who didn't know me well came up. "You would never touch this," she said, gesturing at the feast. I cringed a little and quickly dispelled this idea by letting her know that I'd been eyeing the chocolate peanut butter pie.

People who don't know me make a lot of assumptions about the way I eat, probably because they know food is my area of expertise. That makes sense. But I'm often surprised by their assumptions. They hypothesize that I don't like food or that I'm a strict mouse who only eats salad. I guess that surprises me because what human being doesn't like food? So over and over again, I tell them: "I *love* food. It makes me happy. What makes me unhappy isn't food. It's when *I* eat too much of it. Or too little. That's what makes me unhappy." And that is the truth.

It's likely the same for you. It's not chocolate-chip cookies that ruin your day. It's when you eat five of them and find yourself deep in the throes of regret that causes you grief.

Food makes me happy in all kinds of ways. It tastes good—so amazingly spectacular. I spend my free time looking up new restaurants, food reviews, inventive recipes, and cooking videos. Next week, I am going to Charleston for the first time. The very first thing I did after making plans to be in the city was look up restaurant reviews and make a list of the best options. In fact, my favorite thing to do in new cities I visit is schedule a food tour. Almost every city has one. A guide walks you around the city taking a bite of food here and there at different well-loved restaurants. Often, the foods they choose have a historical significance to the city. For example, I mindfully tasted beignets in New Orleans and Detroit-style pizza when in Michigan. I even like to watch food being made when I don't get to eat it: in the past few years, I've been mesmerized by internet videos that show just hands, at fast speed, making recipes.

Most of all, I love to enjoy great food at home. My husband and I have friends, parents of our kids' friends, who love to cook. They bring over their creations, and my family gets to be the guinea pig—lucky us! Yesterday, they brought a vegan strawberry, blueberry, and blackberry crisp with a brown-sugar-sprinkled crust. We spend Friday nights making food together, drinking wine, and chatting. I can't even tell you how happy that makes me.

I love the taste of my favorite flavors on my tongue and expanding my palate. This year, for example, when traveling in Sicily, I ate a prickly pear for the very first time. I remember looking at it closely. The green skin was bumpy and unfamiliar to me. I didn't even know how to eat it. Thankfully, my friend showed me how to slice it and take a bite—seeds and all. It was sweet and different—unlike any other fruit I have had. Now it's added to my list of dessert items that I enjoy.

Think for a moment right now. What about food makes you happy? Trying new things? The taste? Sharing food with friends? There are just so many aspects of food to love.

Still, it's not just the deliciousness of food that makes me joyous. Yes, that's a big part of it. But here is a confession. I am such a better person when I am well fed and eating mindfully. Maybe you are, too. Well-fed Susan is much more patient with her kids. She doesn't let their minor squabbles bother her. She can wade through tasks she doesn't enjoy as much, like paying bills or paperwork. The not-hungry, mindfully fed Susan is very present mentally. She can listen to your story in counseling or on the phone and remember every single word of it. On the other hand, the empty-stomached version of Susan misses details because that nagging little thought, "What should I eat?" keeps popping into her mind, distracting her.

I'm at my best when I'm like a mindful-eating Goldilocks: I don't have too much or too little, but something that's just right. I love the feeling of having eaten just enough—satisfied, but not too full.

"One cannot think well, love well, sleep well, if one has not dined well," Virginia Woolf wrote, close to a hundred years ago. It's one of my favorite mantras in life, and I include it in all my writing. And my goal is to help people do just that. But what I have found for myself, and others, it is that it takes some very specific strategies to make that happen. It's not easy, but possible!

---

10 Types of Hangry People

Not all hangry people are the same. In this chapter, we will review all the reasons people get hangry. And all the ways they express it. But as I've seen people in my office talk about hanger, year after year, I've discovered some interesting common themes.

The bottom line: all hangry people suffer from a chronic mismatch between their hunger level and the actions they take to satisfy it. To prevent hanger, you have to get to know your hunger like the back of your hand. So as you read these examples, think about how they can help you be mindful of your own hunger.

After you read, take a moment to pause and ask yourself if you identify with one or more of these types (you can be more than one).

1. Too Busy to Eat

Each morning, Karen packs lunches for her three kids and struggles to find their socks and get homework into backpacks, all while trying to choose the right pair of shoes for her own morning meeting. "I want to eat healthy," she says, again and again. But those words are always

---

followed by "but I just don't have time." To Karen, eating feels like a time luxury she can't afford.

The consequence: When Karen gets to work, she rummages around the office looking for anything she can find, usually stale muffins in a meeting room or a Diet Coke at her desk. The majority of the time, she runs on empty. At work, she's grumpy, unfocused, and often thinking about lunch hours ahead of time.

2. Too Little Routine

Thomas installs drywall. Every day, he goes to a new house. And every day, the job is different. Some jobs last an hour. Others last all day. When jobs run long, Thomas works diligently through lunch.

The consequence: By the time he leaves at the end of the day, Thomas is hangry. When he gets home, he stomps in the door and is grouchy toward his wife and kids. And then his wife gets annoyed at him for ruining his appetite by snacking while she's preparing a healthy dinner.

3. Too Much Trouble

Kristina's husband works three evenings a week. On nights he is home, she plans a healthy meal for the two of them. But when she's alone, she thinks: "Make a meal just for me? That's too much effort." Instead, she eats a bowl of cereal or a few handfuls of microwave popcorn and calls it a night.

The consequence: Kristina goes to bed hungry or unsatisfied. The next morning, she wakes up starving. And that sets off a negative cycle of eating for the whole day.

4. Too Hard to Diet

Sarah is trying to lose twenty pounds of post-baby weight. She's tried multiple diets. Some fad diets work in the short term, but she winds up putting the weight back on. Now, she starts her day with coffee, hoping it will curb her appetite for the morning.

The consequence: By lunchtime, she's starving, so she gives up and overeats. Every day, she promises herself she'll eat better, then finds herself in the same pattern by noon the next day.

5. Too Much Mindless Eating

During daytime hours, Jill looks like the model of perfect health. But around ten at night, when her husband goes to bed, she gets bored and feels the need to unwind from a stressful day. She reaches for a bag of chips or bowl of ice cream and snacks on anything salty or creamy.

The consequence: Jill has trouble sleeping because she feels guilty about overeating, which sets her up for a tough day—and more snacking the next night.

6. Too Few Nutrients

Rachel is an elder-care nurse who drives from home to home to visit her clients. Between visits, she fuels up on whatever is easy to pick up in her car: candy, fast food, or a package of cookies from the grocery store.

The consequence: Rachel's body is running exclusively on sugar and processed food. Her body is getting no real nourishment. The spikes in her insulin level all day long lead to intense ups and downs in her mood.

7. Too Much Change

Joel works at a giant clothing store, unpacking shipping crates from sunup to lunchtime. The tough labor takes a huge amount of energy and calories, so he eats a lot to keep from being hangry at the end of the day. But on the weekends he spends most of his time on the couch. He can't figure out how to adjust his eating on weekends.

The consequence: Joel sometimes eats too much on the weekends, when his body doesn't need as much energy. And sometimes he eats too little at work, trying to make up for the weekends. His body is in a constant state of confusion, always trying to run on too little or deal with too much food.

8. Too Confused

"I could eat any time of the day," Mary says. But that's very different than being hungry. Years of dieting have completely warped her understanding of her hunger cues. She can eat until she feels stuffed but still has trouble stopping if the food is tasty.

The consequence: She's not sure she can even tell the difference between genuine hunger and a craving that she can satisfy without going overboard.

9. Too Social

Laura and her husband have been married for five years. "He doesn't have to worry about his eating," she says. "And I gain weight just by looking at food." But her husband's food choices actually have a big effect on hers. When her husband snacks at night, she snacks. If he skips breakfast, she tends to skip breakfast, too. And it's not just her husband's choices that affect her. At work, if her friend orders a salad for lunch, so does she.

The consequence: Laura's food choices don't have anything to do with her own hunger or needs, so they leave her feeling unsatisfied or overstuffed—and hangry.

10. Too Stressed Out

Wendy is recently divorced and has a child with severe autism. Between bills and unexpected episodes with her son, each day brings new challenges. Worry keeps her from sleeping well, and she's got little patience with people at work who complain about little things, when her life is so full of real problems. Sometimes she's so stressed out, it kills her appetite. Other times she overeats to soothe her nerves.

The consequence: The ups and downs in her sleep and eating are starting to show as her weight creeps up, her health plummets, and her hair begins to gray.

CHOOSING HAPPY VS. HANGRY

Growing up, I loved Choose Your Own Adventure books. They were a series of children's books in which you get to decide the next step of the main character in the book, by making a choice at the end of each page: Do you want to run out of a cave because you're afraid of dangerous animals? Then you turn to a certain page of the book. Do you want to continue into the cave, searching for treasure? Then you turn to a different page. This is very different from most traditional books, in which you follow along with the plot and have to go where it leads you, whether or not you like the ending. In the Choose Your Own Adventure series, you take a much more dynamic role, with active choices.

Unfortunately, in many ways, we treat our eating choices like traditional books, just seeing where things go. We feel powerless to change the plot. But I believe eating can be more like one big Choose Your Own Eating Adventure. You have the power to choose where you end up: how your eating will evolve, and how that will affect your mood.

Every day, we have all kinds of opportunities (#hungertuni ties or #hangrytohappy) to pick foods that turn our hunger into happiness. Every time we eat, we choose between happiness and hanger. And hanger isn't something that happens only *before* we eat. We can also feel moody *after* we've eaten things that don't really satisfy us or that fill us up too much. But whether it happens before or after we eat, hanger is the opposite of happy: feeling content with and sustained by our food choices. Happiness, for me, isn't really smiling and feeling joyous. It's a feeling of contentment and satisfaction.

Whenever I eat, I ask myself a simple question: *Will eating this right now bring me hanger or happiness?*

It's a question I hope you'll start to ask yourself, too.

Let me give you an example. This morning, I opened the refrigerator, coffee in hand. "Okay, what's for breakfast, Susan?" I asked myself. Then I ran through my options: everything from a premade smoothie to some dry cereal. I knew I had a big day ahead of me. Clients that needed me to focus on them. A staff meeting. Soccer practice for my kids.

I like a lot of different breakfast foods. So my question wasn't what would taste good to me.

It was "What will make me happy, not hangry?"

When I ask that question, instantly the conversation changes in my head. I start to think about the foods that will fill me and keep my energy up and prevent me from getting hangry, which can happen so easily when we're busy. At the end of the day, it's a chicken-and-egg experience. Which comes first in the hanger spiral, not eating well, or being hangry? It's hard to tell, because not eating well leads to hanger and being hangry leads to not eating well.

My guess is that you picked up this book because you know all too well the downsides of not feeding yourself mindfully. Maybe you haven't eaten enough and withered into a not-so-nice version of yourself. Or maybe you ate too much and turned into someone wracked by regret, guilt, and irritation—at yourself, most of all. Maybe, like most people, you've had both experiences.

I won't promise you that there's a magic bullet for eating mindfully 100 percent of the time. From working with hundreds of clients, I know that's not true. And I know it from trying to manage my own hunger myself. You won't find any magic bullets in this Hanger Management system. Instead, it's a set of strategies and a way of being. It's built to help in any scenario. And it works!

We'll begin by understanding hanger—the science behind it: psychological, biological, and social. Once you learn the roots of hanger, you'll get to know how hanger affects *your* life directly. Is it something that you struggle with only now and then? Or do you fret about your hunger level every day? Understanding how hanger affects you is the jumping-off point for the rest of the book: the tips that can help you deal with hunger in all kinds of situations.

As a busy professional and parent, I know that time is of the essence for my clients. Like you, they're already busy. They don't want to add anything extra to their day. So the tools I've developed to help them eat more mindfully are quick and easy to grasp, even for someone with the busiest of schedules. This book is designed so that you can crack it open and find relevant strategies in just moments.

And when you finish this book, this is my wish for you: I want you to understand that hanger is a real issue that impacts your life on so many levels that it deserves your attention. I want you to stop blaming yourself for not eating mindfully, as if it's a personal failure. You will see that it isn't. And I want you to have the mindful-eating tools to manage your hunger into happiness.

Hanger's a big deal. Bigger than a lot of us realize or want to admit.

But the good news is that we can do something about it.

It's in our hands.

It's up to us to choose.

Part I

HANGER MANAGEMENT 101

From Hangry to Happy

I don't have to tell you that hanger can damage your life. Some of the trouble is subtle. All of us know what it's like to feel distracted or foggy because we haven't eaten well. But hanger can also affect our lives in major ways we may never have realized. Hanger can dull decision-making and kill our mood in important moments. Left unchecked, it can sabotage relationships, both at home and at work. Most of us have firsthand experience of this. And the research backs it up. The science just emphasizes why it is so important to turn hanger around—to make turning it into happiness a high priority. I've heard it a million times—clients who explain why they have a hundred other things that are more important than managing their hanger. But I think the research will make you think twice—it definitely made me give it a spot high on my priority list!

HANGER FREE = HAPPIER RELATIONSHIPS

Where does hanger cause the most trouble, according to studies? One of the most notable research articles on hanger, and one of the first studies I encountered that really piqued my interest, shows that hanger poses the biggest threat to our closest relationships.[1]

When I read this study from Ohio State University, I was intrigued. For one thing, it was the first study I had ever read that used voodoo dolls! For another, it focused on married couples. (That's unusual in research, which is done most often on rats or college students.) And the study took a very practical look at something that happens every single day.

The study was simple. For twenty-one days, researchers measured glucose levels in 107 married couples. But they also gave the participants voodoo dolls meant to represent their spouse. To measure aggressive impulses, researchers asked the participants to stick pins in the voodoo doll each night if they were frustrated with their spouse. Participants could also blast their spouse with loud noise via headphones. The study found that participants who had lower glucose levels stuck more pins in their voodoo dolls. And they also blasted their spouse with louder, longer doses of noise.

I wondered if this research was a little extreme. It's one thing to poke a voodoo doll with pins, but it's another thing to hurt your partner with sharp words that hurt their self-esteem or push their buttons. So I started informally asking people, "Has hanger ever affected your relationship?"

The first response I got was from my friend JT. He wrote:

Is "hangry" a real thing?

In my experience, YES.

I once dated a woman who was very sweet and considerate to all those who crossed her path. She patiently dealt with many of my quirks and flaws on a daily basis.

All of those admirable qualities vanished as soon as her hunger set in. She would change into a hangry person who I did not want to be around and a person who she did not want to be.

Two months into our relationship, we had a nice emotional connection and there were real possibilities of a long-term commitment.

Then, early one Sunday afternoon, she arrived at my house hungry. And very quickly became hangry.

I offered to take her out to eat. As soon as she got in the car, I got the silent treatment and glaring looks, as if I was an idiot for not owning a helicopter that could get us there faster.

Then we arrived at the restaurant. There was a twenty-minute wait for a table.

"Where else do you want to go?" I asked. "I'll take you."

"I don't know," she said. "Wherever you want."

With the pressure on, I picked another place that we'd been to before and both liked. When we parked, I could see they were not busy and we could be eating within fifteen minutes. Hallelujah! But before we got out of the car she said, "I'm not in the mood for anything they have."

Now with two strikes against me, I needed to feed this woman fast. I was sweating. I was terrified to speak.

We sat in the car and I proposed options.

How about the pasta place? "No. I've never been there."

How about the Cajun place? "I don't like spicy foods."

Any place you can think of that you like? "No."

At that point, I remembered what I was doing before she came over. I was happy. It was the weekend. The weather was nice. I was ready to hang out at home and watch the game. Life was great.

Now visibly frustrated and angry myself, I made the call to go to a carry-out sandwich shop.

We made it back to the house without further incident. She ate. I said nothing.

Then she started crying.

She apologized and said she never wanted to treat me like that again. She said hanger had been something that she always dealt with.

But I could not forget. Mostly because it happened several more times. I worried about a long-term commitment with someone who may unleash that behavior after a missed meal or slow service at a restaurant.

We went on to date for a year. We broke up for several reasons, most of which had nothing to do with her hanger. But when I think back, it was a factor. Should a significant other be subject to that kind of treatment just because someone is hungry? Absolutely not.

We often think about how a rumbling in our stomach impacts ourselves. We don't think as often about how our eating impacts those around us. But at the end of the day, how we take care of ourselves has a huge ripple effect on those around us.

I'm sorry for what I said when I was hangry…

My client Brooke was wedding-dress shopping with her sister Jackie, who had flown in from Chicago to help Brooke find the perfect gown. It was going to be a marathon day: Jackie was in town only Saturday, flying out the next day. So they had made back-to-back appointments at three of the most glamorous shops in the city.

In each shop, Jackie ran back and forth tirelessly from the fitting room to the front of the store, fetching dress after dress. Brooke tried on every version of her dream gown—an A-line with an empire waist. And at the last shop, they found it: the perfect dress.

The sisters returned home victorious but exhausted. They melted into Brooke's living-room chairs and began to chat about old times and Jackie's vision for her bridesmaid's dress. Jackie started to reminisce about how their mom used to dress them when they little. The two girls weren't twins, but they were only eighteen months apart, so their mom had dressed them identically until they were old enough to pick out their own clothes.

It might have just been a pleasant walk down memory lane, but then the conversation made a quick, unexpected turn. Tears began to roll down Jackie's cheeks. "You were so selfish," Jackie told Brooke. "Always taking my clothing. You were the favorite child. You got all the best clothes. Mom loved to take you shopping."

Because Brooke is a great sister, she fell silent for a moment. And she thought, Was this conversation really about their clothing options at age four? No, Brooke realized. This was the powerful effect of hanger. She had seen firsthand the difference in her sister before and after eating well, in many emotional episodes. Also, Brooke felt ravenously hungry herself.

Brooke didn't want to engage Jackie's negative ideas and make things far worse. They had just had a great day. And she knew she had a very small window of opportunity to change the direction of this conversation.

So she looked at her sister and simply said, "Let's get something to eat. I think we're both tired and cranky."

Brooke headed straight for her fridge, flung it open, and rummaged through quickly. Then she ran over to her sister with a yogurt like she was a medic delivering an IV at an emergency scene. They each had a cup of yogurt. Before she knew it, Hangry Jackie had disappeared—and Brooke was in a better mood, too.

With each bite, Jackie started to perk up and feel like herself again. And the fun version of herself came back—the one that had just enjoyed her day laughing and being her sister's stylist.

Once she got something to eat, Jackie apologized for the

words that had spilled out of her mouth. She admitted she had felt a wave of hanger coming on. But she hadn't realized that shopping is a big culprit in hanger, because it's surprisingly active and exhausting.

"I should have taken a break between shops two and three," Jackie confessed. "Then I wouldn't have wilted into an emotional mess at home."

The two sisters learned a few things from this incident. Next time, fuel up before an intense shopping experience. Also, eat well before you talk — particularly on an emotional day.

And they put those lessons to work in the wedding itself. Jackie decided that it was really important for the entire wedding party to fuel up the morning of the wedding, to prevent tempers from flaring. Weddings are times of high emotion to begin with, and they didn't want to risk a family hanger session, due to some old extended family drama that could spark at any moment.

They couldn't control everything about the big day. But they could help everyone start with a well-nourished stomach. So Jackie planned a protein-filled breakfast before the ceremony and some filling snacks between the ceremony and the reception, during pictures. The wedding went off without a hitch.

And today, the sisters laugh together about the hanger incident — thankfully.

What's Going On in the Background?

"When my husband is angry," my client Melanie told me, "he has no qualms about taking it out on me." And it isn't just her. When her husband is in the throes of hanger, everyone in a fifty-foot radius knows it. Melanie tries to be more sensitive during those times. But he doesn't return the favor. When she's not well fed, he chalks her behavior up to her being "difficult," rather than dealing with hanger. This bothers Melanie, a lot.

"Why is he like this?" she asked me.

My thought: some people, due to their upbringing, may be more likely to air their grievances and more comfortable expressing aggressive behavior when they are hangry. Some of my clients, like Melanie, come from homes in which conflict is extremely taboo: a single cross word might result in the silent treatment. When people from that kind of background get hangry, they feel guilty and often stuff down those angry feelings or take out their aggression in private and secretive ways. Melanie doesn't lash out at all directly when hangry. She has a secret file of notes that she writes—page after page of angry thoughts. This file contains candid and unedited thoughts that she literally keeps locked away.

But another client of mine, originally from New York City, comes from a "no filter" family, and has been cited by the police for road rage. When he is hangry, he doesn't hold back a bit, including flipping people off on the road or yelling curse words. The difference between these two clients is not simply their level of hanger. It's also at least partly the result of the personalities, family backgrounds, and cultures that shape how comfortable they are expressing negative emotions.

HANGER FREE = BETTER DECISIONS

Hanger doesn't just sabotage our relationships. Researchers have also found that hanger can drastically affect our decision-making skills. Consider this: a prisoner's chance of getting out of jail may hinge on whether a judge is hungry or not.

In a study of Israeli courts, Jonathan Levav and his colleagues at Columbia Business School analyzed 1,112 parole hearings, presided over by eight judges over a ten-month period.[2] The judges' days were divided into three sessions, and each session had breaks for meals or snacks. The judges chose when to adjourn for their breaks, but they didn't control the type of cases they saw or the order in which they saw them.

At the beginning of a session, a prisoner had a 65 percent chance of being paroled. This declined to almost zero by the end of a session, and leapt back to 65 percent after a snack break. Mental fatigue may account for some of this. When we're tired, we go back to the decision that takes the least amount of effort. So when a judge gets tired, it may be easier to default to the earlier decision, and deny parole.

But the researchers also suggest that hunger and low blood sugar help create mental fatigue. After a meal, the decisions of the judges dramatically changed. Overwhelmingly, judges appeared to be harsher when hungry. It's scary to think that your fate might hinge on whether a judge took a snack break. And it might give us a hint about when to ask a boss or significant other for a favor— right after lunch! (Don't even think about asking for anything important right *before* lunch!)

Researcher Andreas Glöckner suggests an alternative explanation for the judges' decisions.[3] He believes that judges may give harsher sentences because they tend to schedule simpler cases in the morning. They do this because more complicated, lengthier cases run the risk of running over into the lunch break.

At the end of the day, we won't know for certain what causes judges to make harsher rulings. It's likely a complex set of reasons. But one thing is clear—it certainly isn't advisable for judges—or anyone—to make important decisions on an empty stomach. I personally would not want to be standing in front of a judge right before lunch—would you?

In a meta-analysis of forty-two studies related to the effect of low blood-glucose level on thinking, researchers examined four dimensions of decision-making. They looked at willingness to pay, willingness to work, impatience, and decision style. They found that low levels of blood glucose, or being hungry, increased the willingness to pay and willingness to work when a situation is food-related. In other words, people will do whatever it takes to get food when hungry — pay big bucks or put some effort into the task at hand. However, when the task didn't have anything to do with money, hunger made people less willing to pay or work in all other situations. For example, if you were at a store and hungry, you would be less likely to exert any effort to look for a different size or pay a high price for a shirt you wanted. Also, when people have low levels of blood glucose, they became more impatient with decisions about food but less so with decisions about money.

Low levels of blood glucose also increase the tendency to make more intuitive rather than deliberate decisions about food. We know this! This is the problem. When hungry, we don't stop to mindfully think it through, we grab the first thing in sight. The overall gist is that low blood sugar affects decision-making, most notably about food decisions.

Another reason not to make an important decision when you are hungry is ghrelin. Ghrelin is a hormone that is released before meals, known to increase appetite. It has a negative effect on both decision-making and impulse control. To understand its effects better, researchers looked at the impact of raising ghrelin levels in rats. They found that when they increase ghrelin levels to mimic levels when rats (and people) are hungry, the rats are more impulsive. The rats had been trained to earn a reward by not pressing a lever. But when ghrelin levels were high, they had much more significant difficulty restraining themselves — even though it meant they lost the reward.[4] Our impulsive decisions and actions are never our best ones.

HANGER FREE = BOOSTS YOUR BRAIN POWER

"I'm taking the ACT tomorrow," a high school student, Becky, said to me. *"I am so stressed about the test and the impact the scores could have on my future plans to be a physical therapist. I will be sure to get a good night's sleep and a really solid, healthy breakfast."*

I happen to know that Becky skips breakfast almost every single day. So I paused and inquired why she planned to eat a healthy breakfast. Without skipping a beat, she said, "I will likely focus much better."

I had to gently point out the irony of this situation. Becky fully realized the importance of a good breakfast on one particular day. She wouldn't dream of going into that test hungry or not well fed. The connection in her mind was extremely clear. Breakfast = better focus. But doesn't it matter if she focuses well on ordinary days? Each week, Becky took tests in school that were important to her future. She made decisions that needed her full attention. Why did it seem worth the effort that day, but not every other day?

Becky laughed when I said all this.

"I hadn't thought of it that way," she said.

It's not just Becky. The effect of hanger on the brain is especially strong in many kids at school. A recent Cambridge University review brought together multiple studies with one thing in common: they all showed that kids who don't have a solid breakfast don't do as well at school. Without breakfast, kids' cognitive skills, mood, and mental sharpness all take a hit, and they actually require more sleep. But unfortunately, 20 to 30 percent of children and adolescents still skip breakfast daily.[5, 6, 7] This is particularly scary given that just eating breakfast helps people remember things and improves their performance on cognitive tests.[8]

A dose of glucose, which we get from food to power the brain, has been shown to help boost recognition memory, visuospatial function (the ability to mentally manipulate two- and three-dimensional objects), processing speed and reaction time, working memory, problem solving, and attention.[9] Wow! These are all things we need to conquer the day!

Most of us could also cite our own "research" on the effects of hanger on our decisions. Time and time again, my clients admit making decisions they regret when they're hangry, from grabbing a quick fix of junk food to making silly mistakes at work and at home. *Urban Dictionary* includes the term "dumb hunger," which they describe as "You are so hungry you can't make a decision" or you make a foolish one, like eating old hot dogs from a gas station or skipping an important meeting to get lunch. Later, you totally regret making that decision.

My client Stephanie refers to her "pineapple dress" with embarrassment when we talk about hunger and decision-making you wish you could do over. In the back of her closet, Stephanie has a hideous black dress with loud yellow pineapples scattered all over it. She bought it to go on vacation in Mexico. It's hung there for many years with the tags still on. She hasn't gotten rid of it, partly because she can hardly believe she would actually buy something so ugly and partly because it's like a warning beacon. She explains that she bought the dress on a shopping expedition while in the throes of hanger. She distinctly remembers thinking, "I don't care anymore. I'm starving—this will do." Have you ever experienced buyer's regret from something you bought during a hangry episode?

And even though I'm a psychologist who deals with hanger day in and day out, I'm not immune to making mindless decisions myself when hangry. Several years ago in California, I gave a lecture on mindful eating. I was the last person up on a panel, and the lectures of the physicians before me went on and on— two hours longer than they were supposed to. When I finally gave my lecture and got out of the room, I realized I was starving! My stomach was rumbling. I had a headache. But I was due to be at another lecture immediately.

Desperate, I opened my purse. I dug to the bottom and discovered a bag of trail mix so old that it was mostly crumbs. I began to ask myself a series of questions that should have stopped me immediately: "How old exactly are these? How did they get in here?"

I remembered that I had packed them weeks ago when I was watching my twin niece and nephew. But then hunger overwhelmed my attempt at personal integration. I gave up and ate every single bit in that bag.

Almost immediately, I regretted it. I didn't enjoy the trail mix. I'd never have eaten kids' old snacks under any other circumstances. And they didn't do anything to help the hunger. A better plan would have been to use what I know. I have been to a hundred conferences. Wordy presenters almost always run over scheduled time limits. I could have armed myself with a good snack in advance.

My clients tell me similar stories, with the same outcome. It always goes like this: getting too hungry results in reaching for whatever is near, whether you like it or not: stale donuts in the break room or baloney in the fridge.

Hanger sends us into scavenging mode. It's a basic biological reaction. But if we don't manage it, the result is regret, frustration, and weight gain/health issues.

At first glance, hunger might seem like a little thing, easy to ignore. And hanger might seem like the punchline to a joke. But as we've seen here, the research is clear: hunger has a dramatic impact on everything from how we react in our relationships to the way we make big and little decisions every day.

HANGER FREE = LESS GUILT

One of the important benefits of getting a handle on hanger is steering clear of the awful feelings that come from overeating. When you are overly hungry, the next meal or snack is frequently not your finest.

"I feel terrible. I wish I hadn't eaten that."

This is the mantra of someone who is in the midst of a "regret-full" state. Being hangry and being regretfull both prompt seriously bad moods. Research indicates that people who overeat or eat particular kinds of foods like treats and chocolate often express shame and guilt.[10]

Unfortunately, even a bit of chocolate can prompt feelings of guilt. Thirty-seven healthy, normal-weight women ate a chocolate bar, an apple, or nothing. They rated how they felt before they ate and 5, 30, 60, and 90 minutes after eating. Both chocolate and the apple reduced hunger, boosted their moods, and increased their energy levels. However, eating chocolate was followed by good feelings for some women and guilt for others.

If eating just a small amount of chocolate causes feelings of regret, you can guess that eating too much chocolate can make you feel very regretfull. It's not just the physical effects of feeling bloated, heavy, and sleepy from an overdose of food. It's the bad feelings that come from not eating in a mindful way. Nothing feels worse than making a decision but then doing the opposite.

The trick is eating just the right amount of chocolate to make you feel satisfied and not letting guilt guide your decisions.

Forgive me for what I said when I was regretfull.

We've looked at the research on what happens when we don't get enough food. But what happens when hanger causes us to eat too much?

My client Kelly described a day on which her husband had gone to a local bakery early in the morning. Being thrifty, he brought the donut special—a dozen. They were her favorite: old-fashioned glazed cake donuts. He knew this; he was thinking about her when he made his selection.

He and both kids each ate a donut before they headed off to work and school, leaving her alone with nine donuts.

"They were just staring at me from the box," she told me. "They were still hot, and it smelled like the entire bakery was in my kitchen." Kelly had fifteen minutes before leaving for work. "I intended to eat only two," she said. "Typically, I'll savor one or two with some fruit."

Kelly got a cup of coffee and ate one donut. It melted in her mouth and tasted fantastic—the perfect sticky, sweet cake texture. Before she knew it, she had eaten a second donut quickly—too quickly. She broke a third donut in half and told herself, "Just one half more." But after eating the half, she broke off a bit more of the leftover half, and then popped the last fourth in her mouth. *It was just another bite,* she reasoned. *So why leave it?*

The donuts were so yummy that she took another one with her for a snack later in the afternoon. But as she drove to work, taking sips of coffee, she found herself nibbling on the donut.

By the time she got to work, she was jittery from coffee and sugar and hyped up, thinking about the presentation she had to give that morning. She could literally feel the tension in her body. And she was kicking herself mentally for having that last donut. Three was pushing it. But she didn't even really *want* a fourth! *How did that happen?* she wondered. She could tell by the way she felt that she'd eaten too much. She didn't feel good at all.

I am a smart woman who makes decisions every day, Kelly thought. *So why couldn't I stick with my decision to have just two donuts?* That question kept repeating in her head. *How could I have let it snowball into four!?*

As she walked briskly down the hall to her office, she could feel her irritation rising. And so could others. Her employees scattered like cockroaches into their own offices, hoping to avoid her. Her dress felt tight, which only added to her bad mood and negative thoughts.

At eleven, her receptionist got out leftovers and heated them up in the microwave. It was Thai food, and as she began to eat it at her desk, a strong smell of curry wafted toward Kelly.

Kelly slammed her hands down on her desk, got up, marched over to her coworker and began to yell. "That food is smelling up the entire reception area!" Kelly bellowed. "How do you expect anyone to work or get anything remotely productive done?"

Kelly's coworker cowered in surprise, then awkwardly grabbed her takeout container and ran to the break room.

Kelly went back to her desk and angrily typed on her computer. But when she took a moment to pause, she felt terrible about the way she had talked to her coworker. Did she really care about the smell of curry? No. She loved it. What she was really feeling was uncomfortable in her body and this tight dress. She was clearly feeling the effects of being regretfull.

As she recounted this story to me, Kelly's mouth clenched tight in embarrassment.

Later that day, Kelly told me, she began to feel better. She went to her coworker and apologized. She told her that she had been having a bad day but that it was no excuse for the way she had talked to her.

The experience gave her a glimpse of the very powerful effects of feeling regretfull. "That version of me is bad-tempered, testy, irrationally grumpy, and ridiculously easily annoyed," she told me.

And that version of her didn't just show up at work. Her family had experienced it, too. Most of the people around Kelly had taken her hanger outbursts personally, because they had no idea her rants were linked to how she was feeling about her food choices and body.

The good news is that the story ends well. Kelly tried the Hanger Management techniques in this book. She learned how to make decisions about how many donuts to eat—and to stick with them. Most of all, she learned to enjoy everything she ate mindfully, with no regret.

Alas, hanger doesn't come only from not getting enough to eat. As shown in Kelly's story, eating too much can leave people feeling just as uncomfortable and unhappy as they do when they don't eat enough. My clients sometimes even confess very negative things, like "I HATE myself when I overeat. I just feel disgusting all the way around."

Some of the irritation comes from the physical effects of overeating: feeling bloated or overfull. But we also feel irritated by the sense of being out of control. No one likes to make a decision, then not stick with it. And our disappointment with ourselves can snowball into feelings that we typically get when we don't follow through on something—guilt, regret, and shame. The

Hanger Management program aims to help people conquer all of these feelings!

Whatever form hanger takes, whether it's eating too much or too little, this chapter has spelled out that it doesn't do us any favors.

Think for a moment about how hanger impacts you. Which part does it sway the most? Your decisions? Your relationships? Does it make you irrationally angry or keep you from thinking clearly?

Now consider, on the flip side, how eating mindfully could improve your life. Take a minute and really imagine the benefits that would come from being hanger-free. What would be different for you if you ate the way you wished? Do you like what you see? If so, keep reading!

Understanding Hanger: Where It Comes From — and Why

Why is it so easy to lash out at people we love or get downright angry over little stuff, just because we're hungry? And why do we try to grind through the day, ignoring our hunger, when we could easily grab a simple, healthful snack? What is *really* going on inside? Why does hunger create wild mood swings?

The very simple, basic answer is that when we're hungry, our blood sugar drops—sometimes dramatically. And low blood sugar can make us more aggressive. It's a normal, natural biological response. In caveman times, becoming more aggressive when hungry was a good thing. It prompted you to jump in and fight a pack of animals or other humans for your share of a meal. Back then, hangry people were often more likely to survive. But these days, as you will learn soon, hanger is much more complicated than a drop in blood sugar: it is a complex interplay of hormones, various functions in the body, and psychology.

4 Types of Hunger That Can Turn into Hanger

A rumbling belly isn't always at the heart of why we eat. We get the sensation of hunger for different reasons, sometimes physical and sometimes not. Various kinds of hunger trigger different types of hanger. And they require different strategies to manage.

So it's important to understand what kind of hunger you're dealing with—before it turns to hanger.

Health Hunger. This is physical hunger: you haven't eaten for a long time, so your stomach starts to grumble. You get tired. When you don't eat enough, don't eat well, or overeat, your body will let you know. These fall under the *biological* reasons we eat.

When Health Hangry, You Feel: Irritable and angry

When Health Hangry, You Think: "I'm starving. Get out of my way, I need to eat something!"

Head Hunger. This hunger starts in your head. Sometimes hunger isn't physical; it's mental. We often think of this as a craving. You start thinking about the chocolate-chip muffins in the next room. Or all you visualize all day is hot, New York–style pepperoni pizza.

When Head Hangry, You Feel: Desire for something very specific, not just nourishment in general. If you don't get it, you feel deprived or disappointed.

When Head Hangry, You Think: "I just really want it."

Heart Hunger: This hunger has an emotional trigger. It may be a positive emotion like joy that you want to keep going. Or it could be a negative feeling such as stress, anxiety, or boredom, that you want to dull with food. Either way, this hunger doesn't come from physical need, but emotion.

When Heart Hangry, You Feel: An urge for temporary comfort or escape from negative feelings. But satisfying this hanger often leaves you feeling regretful and guilty.

When Heart Hangry, You Think: "I *need* chocolate."

Hands Hunger: This hunger isn't physical. It's triggered by boredom and seeing food within reach. The sight and smell of the food kicks off a sensory response. For example, you smell amazing cinnamon rolls as you walk by a store. Or you see a case of beautifully displayed chocolate crinkle cookies in the break room at work. All of a sudden, you get the munchies. You just want the sensation of crunching on something. But it's only because food is within reach. It's not real physical hunger.

When Hands Hangry, You Feel: Your senses perk up. Your whole body reacts, salivating, sniffing the aroma, or staring at the food. Your hands automatically reach for the food because it stimulates your senses — or just because it's there.

When Hands Hangry, You Think: "But it's right here in front of me. And it looks and smells amazing."

3 BIOLOGICAL REASONS PEOPLE GET HANGRY!

If I had a magic wand, one of the many things I would do would be to poof away the critical words people say about themselves and their eating. Things like, "How could I have been so stupid to eat that? I didn't really want to." Or "I knew I shouldn't have ordered another brownie. I am an idiot."

I don't have a magic wand to make this happen. But I do have some pretty solid information that shows hanger is *not* usually a personal failure. More often, it's a result of pure biology!

When you think about what is going on below your skin, you begin to understand why hanger happens so often and why it is important to stay ahead of it. Hanger is a totally normal and natural response, driven by a number of biological factors. Here, I will explain three of the most prominent ones: imbalances in your blood sugar, the stress hormone cortisol, and a pesky neuro-peptide that impacts your desire to eat.

1. Blood Sugar Imbalances

The first trigger of hanger is a fluctuation in blood sugar, also known as blood glucose. When you eat, your body takes the macronutrients from food—proteins, fats, and carbohydrates—and breaks them down into smaller compounds—mostly amino acids, fatty acids, and simple sugars. These compounds are then distributed throughout our bodies to give us all the energy that powers everything from basic needs, such as breathing, to more intense activities, such as running six miles or taking an exam. When you haven't eaten in a while, your blood-glucose levels dip and your body isn't getting what it needs to function well.

Since glucose is the main energy source for our body, it's easy to see how a lack of it can lead to fatigue, irritability, and trouble concentrating—especially when you're still trying to burn through a busy day. The longer we wait between meals, the less glucose circulates in our bloodstream—and the less fuel our body has to function. It's like trying to run a car without any gas.

The brain works best when it is fed, because it needs glucose to function. But it isn't just the amount of glucose that's important. Where the glucose comes from matters, too. Consuming chocolate or a cupcake leads to a sudden surge of energy-boosting sugar. But it doesn't last long. That's because the simple sugars found in chocolate and cupcakes release glucose into the bloodstream very quickly. They provide around twenty minutes of alertness. Then the sudden, high level of sugar runs its course, our blood-glucose levels crash, and we can be left anxious and unable to focus.

RUNNING ON EMPTY

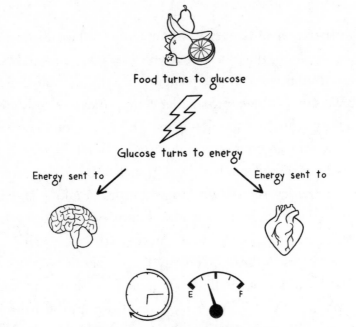

Food turns to glucose

Glucose turns to energy

Energy sent to

Energy sent to

Time passes = Glucose levels drop

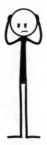

Low glucose = Brain power falls
Difficult to concentrate & focus
Simple tasks become harder and take longer
Cranky
Irritable
Glucose too low = The brain can start to interpret
this as a life-threatening situation

READY FOR BATTLE

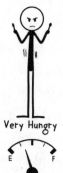

Very Hungry

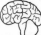

Blood-glucose levels drop
This triggers brain to send instructions to

Synthesizes and releases hormones into bloodstream-
called glucose counter-regulatory hormones

Adrenal gland releases two hormones:

Adrenaline

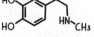

Adrenaline, which increases
aggressive behavior

Cortisol

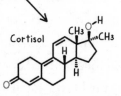

Cortisol, which triggers the
"fight or flight" response

Increase in these hormones
Aggressive behavior
Snappy
Irritable
Confrontational

But when we eat slow-acting carbohydrates, such as fiber-rich foods (whole grains, nuts, and berries), the same amount of glucose is released over a much longer period. And that means we feel more energetic and more alert for hours after we eat.

I often think of the blood-sugar process in our bodies as being like the fuel systems in our cars. When the gas tank first starts to run dry, the car sends you a subtle message that you have to be on alert to even notice—the gas gauge is getting low. If you ignore this or don't notice it, the car ups the ante. It dings or turns on a light to get your attention. And if you ignore that, then you might be in real trouble, and even sputter to a complete stop. At this juncture, you are likely desperately searching for a gas station as close by as possible. Or, in the case of your stomach, whatever food is within reach.

2. Survival Mode and Stress Hormones

Blood sugar doesn't just affect our energy and concentration.

When our blood sugar is low, our bodies go into a state of alarm. And because our bodies are extremely intelligent machines, they start turning on a survival mechanism to prevent starvation. What's the survival mechanism? A "backup generator" for glucose.

When our blood sugar drops, we release hormones that tell our own bodies to start making more glucose out of fat and protein—a process called glucogenesis.

First, a hormone called cortisol increases, which kicks off the production of glucose in the liver in order to flood your body with energy. Next, adrenaline jumps, which you can thank for the jittery, sweaty feeling and increased heart rate that sometimes come with hanger. Together, cortisol and adrenaline make the heart work harder, pump faster, and distribute glucose more quickly.

THAT FOOD IS MINE!

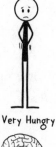

Very Hungry

The brain releases neuropeptide Y

Increases of neuropeptide Y prompt
appetite and feeding behavior

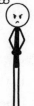

High levels of neuropeptide Y ALSO
increase aggressive behavior

Increase in neuropeptide Y
Biological mechanism encoded to make sure people eat
Intense search for food
Competitive
Aggressive
Obtaining food supersedes social etiquette

When the body or mind is highly stressed, it moves into the fight-or-flight response. It's our body's own protective mechanism, a response to stress in our lives. When we're face-to-face with a bear in the woods, we want all the extra energy we can get. But ongoing stress is too abundant in our modern lives, from work deadlines, family problems, financial issues—you get the picture. We pile on the daily tasks and assume our body will just continue to function as it always has and push us through. But something strange happens to our cortisol levels when we're under constant daily stress. If our stress doesn't go away quickly enough, our cortisol levels can get stuck on "high." When our cortisol levels stay too high, our blood glucose can become permanently elevated. And that has all kinds of consequences: diabetes, high blood pressure, and a weakened immune system.

So hanger isn't just a frustration for us—or the people who have to deal with us. When we ignore our hunger, day after day, it puts our bodies in an ongoing state of imbalance and stress. It doesn't threaten just our mood, but our whole system.

3. Neuropeptide Y

The third major biological process that influences hanger is a chemical that you may never have heard of. It's called neuropeptide Y, and it's a natural brain chemical that is released into your brain when you are hungry and that acts on various receptors in the brain, including one called the Y1 receptor. The result: voracious feeding behavior.

The neuropeptide Y and the Y1 receptors have several jobs. They don't just control hunger. They also regulate anger and aggression. Research has found that people with high levels of neuropeptide Y in their cerebrospinal fluid also tend to show high levels of aggression and impulsive behavior.[11] Understanding this can help us learn to interact with food to cope better with our built-in aggressive tendencies.

As you can see, multiple biological pathways can make us prone to anger and irritability when we're hungry.

But while physical factors contribute to hanger, psychological factors also play a big role.

EMOTIONS = A TICKET TO HANGER

I was in the middle of explaining the biological underpinnings of hanger to my client Julie when she waved her hand and rolled her eyes.

"Yes, that is great and all about my blood sugar," she said. "I'm a wife of a traveling salesman who is never home, a mother of four kids, daughter of a 75-year-old with dementia, and sister to a bipolar brother. That equals about five pounds per person, per year. Which is why I've gained all this weight."

Her point was well taken. Julie's stress level was off the charts. And so was her stress eating.

It's not just our blood sugar that prompts us to overeat mindlessly or not meet our hunger just right. It has a lot to do with how we feel.

I just don't care what the heck I eat. Translation: I feel really angry at myself.

I need to comfort myself with chocolate and sugary treats. Translation: I'm so sad.

I want something to do; maybe I will eat something. Translation: I'm so bored!

I need to gnaw on something. Translation: I need something to calm my nerves.

I lost my appetite. Translation: I'm overwhelmed and stressed.

All of us have powerful emotions, and we're not always sure what to do with them. In our modern world, it's easy to try to lock them away, so we can be more and do more. But when we're out of touch with our emotions, we wind up in whirlpools of confusion and misplaced feelings.

One of the major ways we misplace our feelings is with food. Are we bored? Angry? Anxious? Happy? Too often, we respond to any emotion by eating, or by not eating—even though none of these emotions has its root cause in food. So learning to recognize our emotions and how they're different from hunger is a major step on the path to healthy eating habits.

Maybe you had a really bad day. You're feeling depressed, so you buy a bag of cookies on the way home. Then you eat them with some ice cream you find in the freezer. For a few minutes, you have the thrilling expectation of happiness. But it lasts for all of one bite. Then it turns to disappointment, frustration, and regret.

Or maybe your life just feels too overwhelming. Everything important feels like it's out of your hands. But you know one thing you can manage: how much you eat. Avoiding meals or restricting calories gives you a temporary sense of control, but the aftermath is a downward spiral. And when you can't fend off the body's hangry response, you feel even more helpless than before.

The bottom line: it's not just biology. Too often, we do or don't eat well because of our emotional state. Hanger is caused by a potent blend of biology and psychology. It arises from interactions in all of our systems, mental and physical. And it affects them all, too.

DIETING = ANOTHER DOORWAY TO HANGER

There is a classic, old-school comic strip titled *Cathy*. Cathy, the star of the cartoon, was always on a diet—never successfully, poor thing! Although her cartoons don't use the word *hangry,* she is the epitome of hanger throughout the series. For example, one of the comic strips goes like this: Cathy starts her diet again on Monday. At 9:00 a.m. she vows "to give up sweets." At 9:15 she yells at two coworkers. By 9:20 she eats a donut. As the comic strip runs on, each day after Monday goes just like this. The final frame says, "Three days into my program and all I've succeeded at is cutting out the humans."

It's funny because it's true. Dieters often exhibit a lot of crankiness. They walk into my office and tell me epic tales of hanger. Sometimes they joke about it. But most of the time they don't like their mood or who they are when they are dieting.

One of my clients told me a story about watching the women in her office devour a flourless chocolate birthday cake. They were happily laughing and commenting on the rich, dense cake. She admitted to me that the thoughts she had about the women and the cake were so mean that she was surprised by them. She actually wished the cake was full of laxatives because her diet forbade her from having any.

It's pretty clear that diets can wreak havoc with our emotions. If you have been on a restrictive or fad diet, you know this. It's not a personal failure or something wrong with you. It's the impact the diet is having on your body and mind.

Many weight-loss diets involve low-calorie foods that are often very nutritionally poor, such as low-fat products loaded with artificial ingredients and sweeteners. These diets leave you feeling deprived and your body yearning for healthy calories and nutrients.

As we discussed, your brain needs glucose to run well. When you restrict what you eat, your brain may not get enough glucose, so it is hard to think clearly and keep your mood in check. Also, your brain needs certain foods to help it to create serotonin, the feel-good chemical in your brain and other neurotransmitters. So when you limit your food intake, your mood regulation and feel-good chemicals take a big hit!

Add on the stress of trying to stick to an unrealistic diet and feeling inadequate when you can't, and you have the perfect storm for a continuous pattern of hanger. When dieting, just having to make a simple food choice can send you over the emotional edge.

The mood changes and the feeling blue we experience when dieting often put a quick end to our diets. It's simply not worth feeling that way. In my experience as a person and a professional, when you are in a good mood, you want to eat more healthfully and take care of yourself. Over and over again, I share this message: Ditch dieting. Forever. Just eat mindfully.

In this chapter, I provided a brief overview about the different avenues that lead us to what one of my clients calls Hangry Town. It's a place where you don't want to visit often and if you do, you just pass through quickly—ideally, to a better place of feeling satisfied by what you eat. The roots of hanger are heavily linked with what is happening in your body on a hormonal and blood-sugar level. But that isn't the whole story. How you feel and if you are dieting can also trigger a hangry state. Hopefully, this chapter made you think about how hanger happens and why it's so tough to get past it.

The Hanger Management Program

The good news is, there's hope for turning around hanger!

As I mentioned in the preface, when I first became aware of the concept of "Hanger Management," I didn't have a name for it. I was the parent of two young toddlers, and I just called it survival. All parents will recognize the drill: every time we left the house, I loaded up my bag with portable snacks like bananas, grapes, and pretzels—anything I could feed my two children at a moment's notice. Why? Because as every parent knows, hungry toddlers are a recipe for a catastrophic meltdown. And a few snacks work like magic to get kids' moods back on track. I didn't realize it at the time, but my two children, Brooke and Jack, were my first Hanger Management subjects.

When my oldest child was born, I was hypervigilant. I watched my new baby daughter closely for early signs of hunger. Sometimes she would dig through my bag, listlessly searching for a snack as she did that day at church. Other times, I could see her beginning to wilt like a flower. Or she'd just become a little fussier than usual. In the beginning, before I got her cues down to a science, it was, frankly, trial and error. I saw the results of missing the mark and letting her get too hungry: meltdown! But letting her snack and graze on food all day wasn't the answer either.

That led to battles at the table, not eating with the family, *and* fussiness.

But the whole process intrigued me, and eventually I learned cues that told me *rush in a snack quick before she gets too hungry!* Most parents of toddlers become world experts at managing their children's hunger. But somehow, managing our own hunger cues is a whole different story.

As a psychologist, I see the same hunger effects in my adult clients that I saw in my toddlers. Being overly hungry can take you from a perfectly rational and happy human being to an illogical schmuck in a few seconds flat. I've witnessed firsthand how people can do catastrophic damage to their relationships with spouses, bosses, and children simply because they are in the throes of hunger, or because eating too much food left them feeling uncomfortable and irritable. Things they would never say when calm — things they might not even mean — slip out uncontrollably. And it's hard to explain to your spouse that you said the meanest thing ever just because you were hangry.

Many of us have heard the word *hanger* thrown around in conversations and jokes. But in this book, what does *hanger* really mean?

Put simply, hanger is what happens when we aren't mindful or in tune with our bodies' cues to eat. But the concept of hanger includes this full spectrum of disordered hunger: neglecting food; emotional eating; craving food; making unhealthy, mindless, or haphazard food choices; overeating; and not getting enough nutrients to feel satisfied with the food we consume.

We're all pretty familiar with the idea that we might get hangry without food. But most of us don't realize that the emotional and physical effects of hanger can persist even after we eat. That's because hanger leads us to crave food, especially processed food,

Hanger Cycle Diagram

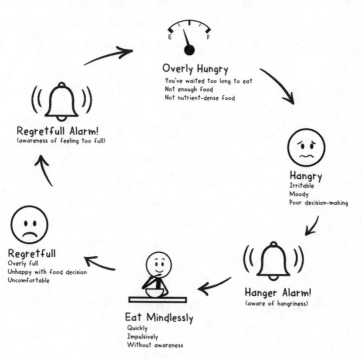

E   F

Overly Hungry
You've waited too long to eat
Not enough food
Not nutrient-dense food

Regretfull Alarm!
(awareness of feeling too full)

Hangry
Irritable
Moody
Poor decision-making

Regretfull
Overly full
Unhappy with food decision
Uncomfortable

Eat Mindlessly
Quickly
Impulsively
Without awareness

Hanger Alarm!
(aware of hangriness)

rich in salt, sugar, and fat, that provides an immediate rush of calories and flavor. These kinds of foods are often easy to find when we're desperate for a quick meal. But since they don't supply your body with the nutrients it's calling for, eating certain food when we're hangry can create a cycle of hanger that can feel hard to break.

On the other hand, eating mindfully has a totally different effect on us. Mindfully choosing foods that give the body and mind the fuel they truly need to function feels good. It gives us greater mental clarity and better emotional stability. In other words, certain foods help our mood, and others make our mood worse.

What I teach my clients is how to tune in and distinguish which foods feel good in *their bodies* and which ones don't. Whatever it is you eat: pizza, candy, or tangerines, it's all great if eaten mindfully. The secret is learning how any food impacts you and your mood.

The big picture advice I give sounds simple enough, and you'll hear it throughout the book. *Mindfully eat food that makes your mind, mood, and body happy and content, not hangry.*

If only this were as easy to do as it is to say. Believe me, I know it's not! But in my daily work with clients, listening to hundreds of stories and delving deep into clinical research, I've found tips and strategies that make mindful eating habits a real possibility.

Hanger Management Diagram

EVERY DAY

Handle Hanger Hijackers
Be mindful of factors that
impact your appetite & hunger

AS YOU EAT

Hack Your Hunger
Pay attention to HOW you eat
Eat each bite mindfully

Satisfied
Content

Hanger-Free Homes & Hangouts
Make a mindful environment to eat

Hunger Hypnotizers
Mindfully choose foods to make your mood & mind happy
Be mindful of how food impacts your energy & mood

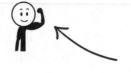

BEFORE YOU EAT

Hear Your Hunger
Assess your:
Emotional vs. physical hunger
Level of hunger
Know & anticipate your hunger cues

I've seen mindful habits change the lives of my clients. They gain energy. They lose and manage weight. They stop emotional eating and develop a better relationship with food. And, as the title of this book promises — they turn their hunger into happiness.

Hanger Management is the series of strategies and techniques that I developed and teach in my virtual practice that are clinically proven to help busy people stay on top of their hunger. It's based on mindfulness, being attuned to your hunger cues, and eating in a strategic way to prevent your emotions from being undermined by hunger. And, much like anger management, it's a system that can change the quality of your life, for the better.

You may wonder why, after writing eight books on mindful eating, I was ready to write yet another book. (Can you tell I love writing books?) It's because I know from my own experience how important managing hanger can be to happiness.

Personally, I first got the hang of mindful eating in graduate school, as I was studying the psychology of mindful eating day in and day out. And, as I taught myself and my clients how to turn on their awareness while eating, I became very attuned to *how* and *why* I ate. But as I went through a transition in my life, a new challenge emerged that made me work on mindful eating again: how could I stay one step ahead of my hunger when I became a parent and a very busy professional? It had been much easier to eat mindfully when it was just me. But when I added new responsibilities to my plate (no pun intended), I had to build mindfulness skills in a new way.

What I realized is that sometimes the stress of parenting was worse when I didn't eat well. And when I did, some of the stress itself could be prevented. I had to find a way to ward off bad moods by keeping my body and mind in good shape so I could deal with the challenges life threw at me. It didn't happen over-night, but eventually I got a handle on how to eat for a healthy, productive life. And you can, too. I've seen these Hanger Man-agement tools and strategies work for all kinds of people, in all kinds of situations.

For example: One day, my coworker came into my office, sat heavily in the chair across from me, and announced, "I'm getting fat." His belly extended over his belt and he began to rub it clock-wise as he told me he was embarrassed to admit he had been struggling to do things that had never been a problem for him before. Simple activities like climbing a ladder to clean the gut-ters at home or holding babies in his medical office were becom-ing harder to do. And he felt like a hypocrite when he told his clients to eat better but struggled to eat well himself.

He didn't like the term *emotional eating*. "My wife calls me a stress eater," he told me. "I do have a stressful job. But I don't do *that*."

"I have a Hanger Management program to tell you about," I told him.

This was a new concept to him. He had heard the word *hanger* before—he even chuckled a little. But he'd never heard of the Hanger Management program before, because that was a term I came up with, to help communicate the idea that there is a sys-tematic way to address our hanger and its consequences.

Right away, his interest was piqued. He liked the idea of a plan. In that moment, everything changed for him.

Together, we discussed the factors that got in the way of man-aging his hunger. It turned out that stress was a big part of it. Fast-forward to today: he's lost the belly. But that wasn't what we focused on. Much more important, he's now much healthier. And even better, he's happier with his energy level and his ability to manage his appetite, even on a stress-packed day. *Food helps rather than hinders his day.*

The strategies I lay out in the five parts of *Hanger Management* changed his life. They have changed the lives of all kinds of people in my clinical practice. And they can help you change your life, too.

One important note. If you continue to struggle while you are doing the Hanger Management program or after, that is okay. Please be sure to contact a qualified health professional. Sometimes you need additional support to unravel these issues, and sometimes there are underlying medical issues involved.

We are not toddlers at the mercy of our hunger-fueled meltdowns. We can recognize our own hunger cues as quickly and effectively as the most vigilant helicopter mom. And we can react to them in a way that keeps us healthy, fit, and happy.

So how does it work?

As you can see in this chart, it's all based on a simple shift: moving from automatic habits to being more mindfully tuned in to the specific cues that tell you when to stop and start eating.

Benefits to Hanger Management

- Increased productivity
- Better decisions and focus
- More stable mood
- Less emotional eating
- Weight loss/management
- Mindful eating
- Better relationships

WHAT YOU WILL FIND IN THIS BOOK
AND THE PROGRAM

What will you find in this book?

Here's a brief overview of each section of the program.

First, you'll notice that each tip begins with a brief question. It's not a quiz with a right or wrong answer. It's just a way to help you to check in with yourself, a way to be mindful. You may notice yourself saying, "Yes, that applies to me. I really need to pay attention to this section." Or you may think the exact opposite: "I've got this tip down pat." No matter which way you answer, it helps to think more deeply about how this particular tip or habit applies to you.

Hangry	To	Happy
No Effort—Mindless		Effort—Mindful
Unconscious		Conscious
Not much awareness of the connection between your daily habits and how they impact your hunger.		**Handling Hunger Hijackers:** Become aware of daily factors that impact your hunger level.
Eating in reaction to triggers in your environment instead of thinking your choices through.		**Hanger-Free Homes and Hangouts:** Arrange your environment to help you eat more mindfully.
Tuning out, over-responding, or under-responding to your hunger.		**Hear Your Hunger:** Listen to your hunger so you can respond to it mindfully.
Not realizing how the food you eat makes you feel or impacts your body.		**Hunger Hypnotizers:** Notice how specific foods impact your mood and body overall.

(continued)

Hangry	To	Happy
Mindless eating, unaware of how food tastes, the impact on your body, your pace, where you eat, and other factors.		**Hack Your Hunger Habits: 10 S's of Mindful Eating:** Be attentive; to break old patterns, enjoy food more and make decisions that you can stick to.
Mindless eating = unhappy, regretfull, unsatisfied.		Mindful eating = happier, content, satisfied.

SECTION ONE: Handling Hunger Hijackers. In the first section, we dive into the factors that **hijack your hunger**. In other words, certain elements set the stage to skew your hunger cues—making them louder or confusing. All kinds of triggers can make us think we're hungry or feel hungrier than we normally would: our environment, lack of sleep, stress, social situations, internal emotions, and so on. To my clients' surprise, many of these factors have absolutely nothing to do with food. They find they have been looking for answers in the wrong places. Their bedroom sleep habits may be more of a culprit in their hanger than what they are putting on their kitchen table.

When Hunger Hijackers act up, hunger triggers can get magnified or dimmed. In this section, we talk about mindful ways to approach each trigger. Although you can easily flip through this book, I often direct people to take a peek at this section first, *before* you start to tackle being more mindful of the way you eat. Just addressing some of these underlying factors may make eating mindfully significantly easier.

SECTION TWO: Hear Your Hunger. In the next section, you'll learn how to really **hear your hunger**. I've found in working with clients that sometimes it is very easy to recognize the signs of hunger. Your stomach gives you some pretty clear signals, like a loud rumbling noise that everyone in a quiet room can hear! But other times, those signals are very subtle and take a particularly close kind of listening to get exactly what your body is saying it needs. But many of my clients have tried to put their hunger signals on mute for years. Turning those signals back on can be tricky, but it's essential to mindful eating. This section shows you how to turn up the volume to mindfully hear what your body needs and then respond consciously.

SECTION THREE: Hanger-Free Homes and Hangouts. Section three is about another powerful way to manage your hunger—**taking charge of your environment**. Your surroundings have a huge effect on what and how much you eat: whether there are healthy or unhealthy snacks in the break room at work, whether you eat alone or with others, and even whether you check your phone during a meal. The shift between eating at home and eating at work is a common area of difficulty. So we'll talk about how to set the stage for a calm eating environment and other ways to create a wonderful haven for mindful eating.

SECTION FOUR: Hunger Hypnotizers. Next, in order to make mindful choices that make you happy, you have to realize that food in general and **certain foods in particular can have a profound impact on your mood**. So we'll talk about what research has found about particular foods and how they impact how you feel. I find this section really interesting. It's not just the quantity of food we eat that can lead to hanger—it's the quality. The body can't be fooled. Remember, and I want to emphasize this so it is loud and clear: **foods aren't good or bad**. We simply need to pay attention to how they impact us and our emotions. When you are mindful of how your body feels and the emotions that kick off after you eat, you notice that you begin to choose food in a more conscious way. When you want to feel a certain way, you will reach for certain foods over others, because you've learned how they affect you.

SECTION FIVE: Hack Your Hunger Habits. Finally, in the last section, we'll dive into how to bring **mindfulness to the table**, with ten easy things you can do to start being more mindful at every meal and snack. I call them the 10 *S*'s of mindful eating. You may want to read all ten of them at once. Or if you feel overwhelmed by all of this information, try reading one a day. For just that day, bring your mindful awareness to one behavior or habit. You don't have to change anything, just notice how this way of eating manifests in your own life.

Managing hunger is never just a matter of rules. We may wish it came down to "Do this, not that!" We may wish that it was simple. But it can be simple when you use your own internal wisdom. This isn't a book about rules. It's about knowing yourself and your own patterns, which are different from everyone else's. So you'll also learn the ins and outs of your individual hunger cues and your personal Hanger Trigger Point. You'll learn to recognize your hunger signals *before* they lead to a hangry disaster. These mindfulness practices will give you a whole new, balanced relationship with food. Remember, Hanger Management is not an isolated dietary approach or fad diet. It's a complete package of realistic, accessible, mindful psychological tools.

Ready?

Let's get started!

Part II

HANGER MANAGEMENT TIPS

Handling Hunger Hijackers

Let's start at the beginning. A great deal of what you eat or don't eat has little to do with what happens the moment you sit down at the table, place your napkin in your lap, and raise your fork. What happens *before* and *after* you eat are just as, if not more, important. Here is an example.

The other day I had a client who arrived an emotional wreck. Crying. Tears. Disheveled. Denise criticized and belittled herself for over an hour about her "awful" food choices that week. The appointment was right after Easter. For days prior to Easter, she stayed up late at night cleaning her house from top to bottom. Her judgmental in-laws were going to be staying the weekend, and she made sure she got every speck of dust out of her house. Easter mass and dinner were lovely. After her in-laws left and the kids were in bed, she tore into their Easter baskets and ate all the chocolate peanut butter eggs she could find. The next day she promised herself no more candy. By noon, she had finished off the rest of the candy in the baskets. She spent the day irritable. "Awful," was the only word she could come up with to describe how she felt physically during and after the onslaught of sugar.

The next week she walked into my office a completely different person. She was calm, smiling, and dressed to the nines. She sat down and breezily said, "I had a great week, no overeating episodes at all." Denise was the picture of Zen.

One might scratch one's head on how one week can be a disaster and the next go off without a hitch.

The week of the chocolate–peanut butter egg debacle, she had been up all night cleaning her house after she had already worked all day at her job as a nurse. I cringed. What I know about Denise is that when she is sleep-deprived, her emotions and ability to make decisions about food make a complete 180. She was just tired. Exhaustion breeds hanger. And proximity to an abundance of chocolate didn't help. This was a very clear example of how certain factors in life, like lack of sleep, can completely hijack your food decisions.

Getting other lifestyle factors into check is sometimes essential to making any changes to your hanger whatsoever. In other words, consider the aspects in this chapter before you dive into managing your hanger so that you create the easiest path possible and know where to invest your efforts.

With Denise, we could have spent all day strategizing about how to avoid Easter candy. Putting it away. Not buying it. Distraction. But, really, getting better sleep was an essential first step to her being able to put all the other Hanger Management techniques into practice. Going to bed earlier wasn't easy for her. Denise is a night owl, often very busy paying bills and doing laundry at night. Making that change took some time and effort but paid off huge rewards in turning her hangriness into happiness.

As you read this chapter, think about how the things that happen before, during, and after you eat impact your food choices.

Consider whether there are things that may be hijacking your ability to make food choices that make you happy and content.

HUNGER HIJACKER #1: TAKE STRESS OFF YOUR PLATE

"When I'm hungry and stressed out, watch out! I just don't care what I eat. Particularly when I have to make a lot of decisions, which I am not good at. Decisions = stress = awful food decisions for me. I say, 'What the hell?' and dive right into whatever's in front of me. Then, I get even more stressed out that I gave in to stress eating when that isn't really what I wanted to do."

When I'm stressed . . .

a) I eat everything in sight.
b) I couldn't care less what I eat.
c) I completely lose my appetite.
d) I promise myself I'll eat better when life slows down — as I dive into that box of chocolate, bag of potato chips, etc.
e) I don't stress eat; I try to do something else to make myself feel better.

No matter which answer(s) you marked, the issue is still the same. Stress doesn't do our appetites any favor.

My client Beth was going through a nasty divorce. Her ex sent her a constant barrage of harassing texts and emails. He couldn't let go. She was so swallowed up in her grief and anger that eating well was the last thing on her mind for weeks. But she was so unhappy with how she felt and was uncomfortable in her body. She described being angry with herself. "Mostly I eat whatever I can find and takes the least amount of effort. It's just me so sometimes I eat cereal three times a day," she said. "Other days, I just want to hide under a blanket and snack on salty chips all night." Finally, after several months, she had had enough of feeling this way.

When Beth entered my office and told me her story and her goal to eat more mindfully, I knew that our first task wasn't to change Beth's diet. In fact, until we changed her stress level, there was no way she was going to eat more mindfully. We couldn't control the ex-husband (though she would have liked to!). But we could work on changing the way she coped with the stress and took care of herself. For many of my clients, we don't even talk about food until we understand the role that stress is playing in their food choices.

The research is clear: stress has a direct impact on your appetite and hunger.[12] And vice versa. Not eating well and being hungry often make you more stressed. And the more stressed we are, the harder it gets to simply take care of ourselves and eat mindfully in the midst of everything else.

Beth was living through a vicious circle that many of us know all too well. When we're stressed, we don't always feed ourselves well. That can lead to hanger, which stresses the body. And when our body is stressed, it's harder for us to cope with any more stress, even small frustrations or annoyances. That's why we're so likely to blow up over little things when we're hungry.

Over time, the constant stress causes chronic inflammation, which starts to play havoc with your body. Have you ever seen a friend age suddenly during a stressful season? Or looked at pictures of American presidents before and after they took office? In a relatively short period of time, they develop wrinkles and strains of gray—often telltale signs of chronic stress.

Study after study shows that when you put people in stressful situations, they have a much harder time making mindful choices about food. In one study, half the participants were asked to dip their hands in icy water, to cause stress. The other half weren't. Then both groups were asked to make choices about food, while their brains were scanned. The ice-water participants, who had just experienced stress, were more likely to choose tasty food rather than healthy food.

Most of us don't dunk our hands in icy water on a daily basis. But the real stressors of life can feel like getting a cold bucket of water thrown on us, out of the blue, time and again: tough divorces, unexpected bills, irritating relatives, frustrating bosses. It's always important not to make any major life decisions when stressed or hungry—doing so often results in poor choices.

Since we can't turn off stress, what can we do?

Dr. Kristin Lindquist, assistant professor in the department of psychology and neuroscience at the University of North Carolina, Chapel Hill, and Jennifer McCormack, a PhD student there, co-authored a study titled "Feeling hangry? When hunger is conceptualized as emotion." They put hungry people in stressful situations to see what would happen. In the study, hungry participants were put into an annoying, stressful situation: a computer malfunction required participants to begin a tedious task over again. You're probably not surprised to hear that participants who were hungry were more annoyed by this computer glitch than those who had a full stomach.

Later, when doing an evaluation of the research assistant's performance, the hungry participants were much more likely to give negative feedback than those who did the study on a full stomach. Bottom line: they could handle stress better when they weren't hungry.

Basically, being hungry and then being in a stressful situation can turn up your irritation level a big notch.[13] However, being mindful or boosting awareness of how you are feeling helps prevent hanger even if you are hungry.

Also based on the research, the authors suggest that we should be *more* aware of our hanger. Let me explain. In the study mentioned above, hungry people who were asked to focus on their emotions were much more likely to attribute being in a bad mood to themselves. But when participants focused on external events, like the stressful computer glitch, they blamed someone else for their bad mood. When participants were aware that they were hungry, they were nicer, less likely to act out on that bad mood. They said to themselves something like, "Hey, I'm really hungry, which is probably why I am in a bad mood." When they had this awareness, they were less likely to act out on that bad mood because they knew why they were grumpy.

The take-home lesson: Tune in. Take a moment to pause, calm down, and assess your hunger level.

Hangry to Happy

Admit to being stressed. When you're stressed, focus on it. That may sound wrong, but people get into regretful situations when they stress eat before they realize they are stressed. It's only after the fact that they realize the true reason they were so out of sorts. So right now, think about how high your stress level is—chronically sky high? Moderate but with brief, acute bursts?

Calm down before you eat. If your stress level is high, remember to pause and ground yourself before taking every bite. Bring the hands-in-freezing-water study to mind, and remember: we make our worst food decisions when stressed. Grounding calms down your fight-or-flight system. And it gets us connected back to the moment. When we're stressed, we're caught in our head in the midst of swirling thoughts. Grounding moves you back into your body, where you can be fully present, aware of your immediate sensations. And you can weave grounding methods right into the meal process. Taking one second to get calm before you eat can help you to make more mindful food choices. Choose one of the following or do all of them.

Plate Grounding. Before you eat, place your finger at the top of your plate. Take a deep breath. Start at the top and run your finger in a clockwise pattern around the plate. Exhale as you do. When you reach the top of the plate, breathe in deep again. Repeat as many times as it takes to feel calmer.

Chair Grounding. When you sit down at a table, place your feet firmly on the floor with your back straight against the chair. Lift both feet at the same time. Hold for a second. Then plant your feet firmly again.

Drink Grounding. Place your hands around your glass for a moment. Tune in to the cold. Observe the glass: maybe it has beads of condensation on it. Release your hands for a moment, then repeat.

Fork & Spoon Grounding. Pick up your fork or spoon. Lightly tap it on the table next to you three times. Listen closely to the sound. Notice how this shifts your focus to the sound, something outside of you. Repeat.

Invest in stress reducers. If you struggle daily with stress, I can't emphasize enough how important it is to invest time and money in stress reducers—a yoga class, a comfy robe to slip into when you get home, relaxing music, a therapy session, movies to distract you, etc. Stop buying diet products, and start purchasing stress reducers! In my book *50 Ways to Soothe Yourself Without Food*, I talk about natural, cheap, and effective ways to relax and destress. They all revolve around calming the sensations in your body so that you exit fight-or-flight mode.

HUNGER HIJACKER #2: SLEEP TIGHT FOR A GOOD APPETITE

"When I get home late from work, I stay up late and get lost down the black hole of my social media accounts. It's hard for me to unwind and turn off my brain. But when I lack sleep, I am completely exhausted. I find myself snacking more, hoping that it will revive me. Sugar or toothpicks seem like a necessity to keep my eyes open at work."

When it comes to sleep . . .

a) I rarely sleep. I'm like a zombie most of the time.
b) I'm usually trying to "catch up" on weekends.
c) I get enough sleep but have bad nights here and there.
d) I prioritize getting at least 7 or 8 hours every night.
e) I get too much sleep.

It's 7:00 a.m. Your eyes are blurry. You tossed and turned restlessly all night. You stumble toward the coffee pot. You are ravenous and have no idea why. You ate a solid dinner.

And when you're feeling this hungry, you don't have to be a fortune teller to predict the likely outcome: hanger is just around the corner.

Sleep deprivation can cause hanger for a whole host of reasons.

At the American Heart Association's Scientific Sessions, one study showed that women who got only four hours of sleep at night ate 329 more calories the next day than they did when they slept a solid nine hours.[14] And another study published in *Advances in Nutrition* concluded that subjects who were sleep-deprived increased their nighttime snacking and were more likely to choose high-carbohydrate snacks.[15] It makes sense that sleep-deprived subjects would naturally go for these foods, since they not only taste good but also make people sleepy. And researchers published in the *Canadian Medical Association Journal* found that people on a diet who slept only five and a half hours a night for two weeks lost 55 percent less fat and were hungrier than those on the same diet who slept eight and a half hours.[16]

The good news? The opposite is also true. Getting more sleep can help us eat more mindfully.

A study recently published in the *American Journal of Clinical Nutrition* found that adults who slept an average of 90 minutes more than their normal sleep time were less hungry and had fewer cravings the following day.[17] In the study, University of Chicago researchers tracked 10 overweight or obese men and women who were in the habit of sleeping an average of 6.5 hours per night or less. During the study, they stuck with their normal sleep routine for one week. But then they increased their sleep—to around eight hours per night for another week. The results revealed that those who went to bed earlier or stayed in bed longer experienced a 14 percent drop in appetite and a 62 percent decline in desire for unhealthy salty or sweet snacks. Wow! That's a lot.

I get a lot of pushback from my clients about getting more sleep. It's not easy. I know. Between hectic lives and the joy one gets from binge-watching TV into the late hours of the night, our sleep schedules are all over the place. And it seems like that's been true pretty much from the dawn of history. In approximately 350 B.C.E., Aristotle wrote an essay, "On Sleep and Sleeplessness." The problem of getting enough sleep has been with us for a long time.

But when we find a way to get more sleep, it has a powerful impact on all parts of our lives—including what we eat.

Hangry to Happy

Don't try to change your sleep schedule right away, I tell my clients.

First, just be more mindful of the role of sleep—or the lack of it—on your mood, energy level, and hanger. Be honest with yourself. When you are low energy due to lack of sleep, do you try to refuel with food? Do you care less about what you eat?

Then, as you're able, begin to try these tips.

Get seven hours—or whatever you need. According to a study on sleep and eating, getting seven to eight hours of sleep per night is optimal for most people. This study found that getting less than 6 hours significantly increases the risk of being overweight or obese.[18] Here is a caveat: Everyone needs their own unique amount of sleep. Some people run well on less than eight hours, and some of my clients need more to even be able to function. Take a moment right now, and think about how much sleep you need and how it impacts your mood and hanger. If you don't know, try writing down how many hours you sleep and your hungriness level over the next few days.

Start small. It doesn't have to be all or nothing. If an extra hour isn't possible, start with something smaller, like heading to bed 15 minutes earlier than normal. Even that small amount has been shown to have a significant impact on your appetite.

Try banana tea. Need help falling asleep? Bananas and their peels have potassium and magnesium to help your muscles and blood vessels relax. Just cut off the two ends of a banana. Place the entire banana, still in the peel, into a pot of boiling water for about eight minutes. Pour the water through a strainer into a mug. Add some cinnamon and, if desired, honey. Drink about four or five minutes before bed. There are more suggestions of foods that can help you get to sleep in Tip # 27.

Get quality sleep. If you struggle with the quantity of sleep, do everything you can to reduce disruptions like pets, light, and noises that reduce the quality of your sleep. Place your phone at least three feet from your head. Better yet, turn off your phone, or at least turn it over. Phones emit blue light and sounds that may impact the quality of your sleep. You can also purchase an app that eliminates blue light!

Find a routine. Routine is your best friend when it comes to sleep. Get to bed at the same time and get up around the same time, as often as you can. And before you go to sleep, use a consistent winding-down pattern that gives you a ritual to calm your body and prepare yourself for sleep, such as a yoga exercise/stretch, saying a prayer, or reading a chapter of a book.

Create a mindful atmosphere. Do you notice that it's hard to sleep when you are too hot? The optimal temperature for comfortable sleep is around 70 degrees Fahrenheit. Also, invest in some quality bedding. People who sleep better in a hotel often realize that the mattress or bedding they are using may be contributing to their difficulty sleeping.

HUNGER HIJACKER #3: LISTEN TO YOUR GUT

Sometimes I feel like I don't know what's going on in my gut. I just know it isn't good. I spend way too much time in the bathroom. Frankly, it's embarrassing. Sometimes I don't even want to go somewhere if I know I'm

*going to have to make a mad dash to the bathroom to relieve the gas gur-
gling in my stomach at any given time.*

When it comes to my gut...

a) I often have a lot of gas, bloating, and constipation.
b) I sometimes struggle with GI (gastrointestinal) symptoms,
   fatigue, and anxiety.
c) I have bloating or gas only when I overeat.
d) I have regular bowel movements, and my stomach usually
   feels fine. My energy and focus are okay.

According to the latest research, your food cravings and mood
may have more to do with your gut than with your stomach.

But what's the difference between your stomach and your gut?

Put simply, your stomach is the muscular organ that helps digest
your food. And your microbiome is the unique combination of
bacteria, hormones, and genetic material that lives in your gastrointestinal tract—the gut—and communicates with your brain.

If you're hungry and/or hangry all the time, the problem may
not be just with your stomach. It may actually be related to
your gut.

When my clients' hunger and appetite are out of whack, I
reassure them that there is a lot going on inside on a microscopic
level. You don't need to blame yourself for the ups and downs,
mood swings, or out-of-control cravings. In fact, studies show
that people who struggle with their weight often have gut bacteria communities that are significantly different from those in
people who don't struggle with their weight.[19]

Hormones in your gut regulate hunger. Your gut may be as
involved as your brain in deciding what to eat. And the delicate

lining of our guts may have been damaged or altered by frequent antibiotic use, sugar, and processed foods that have completely changed or eliminated the helpful bacteria.

It's complicated — but generally your gut hormones also play a critical role in relaying nutritional and energy status signals from the gut to the brain. It's a complex system, full of receptors that release hormones that regulate hunger.

But did you know that your gut microbiome can change for the better in a matter of twenty-four hours? So there's a lot you can do to promote better gut health and optimize your microbiome, as a step to getting your hunger cues back on track.

What is most important for readers of this book to know is that certain foods affect how your gut communicates with your brain, which in turn affects your mood and hanger level. In the last decade, research has revealed an extensive communication network between the gastrointestinal tract and the central nervous system, referred to as the "gut-brain axis." Advances in this field have linked mood disorders to changes in the microbiome. They have found that probiotics, "good bacteria," help people to feel less depressed and anxious.[20] (Note: the strain of probiotic, the dosing, and duration of treatment vary widely in studies.) Wow! This is amazing.

Emmie, my client, has struggled with acne since she was a teenager. Throughout her life, she felt insecure about her random, angry red breakouts. Her self-esteem often plummeted when her skin broke out. Emmie said she often felt anxious in social situations and sometimes refused to go out during an outbreak. She thought her anxiety level was due to years of feeling self-conscious about her skin. And in part, it was. But her doctor had also put her on multiple rounds of antibiotics to treat her skin. While they cleared up her acne, she didn't realize that they destroyed all the bacteria in her body—both good and "bad." That meant that her anxiety level was still really high—and the antibiotics also gave her diarrhea. So she started to be more mindful of how her body felt and added more foods that helped her gut repopulate the good bacteria—which helped her to feel better and less anxious overall and to eat more mindfully.

Hangry to Happy

As part of the Hanger Management program, I ask you to do three things. First, be mindful of whether your gut seems unhappy in some way. Second, if it does, then start being more mindful of foods that make your gut even angrier and more irritated. And third, if you are up for a great experiment, try being more mindful of how your emotions are affected when you eat foods that naturally have probiotics in them.

Listen to your gut. You've heard it before, but maybe not quite so literally: listen to your gut, mindfully. Take inventory of what's going on inside. What is your gut telling you? Is it quiet? Or is it sending you some loud and clear signals that it needs attention?

If your gut isn't complaining, that's a good thing. But if you don't know if your gut is on track, it may be worth experimenting to see if working on your gut health improves your appetite and hanger level.

Certain foods can significantly improve the health of your gut, which puts you on a better path to managing your hanger level. If your appetite feels out of control and you are hungry all the time, getting your gut healthier may help manage your appetite.

Try a gut experiment. Try adding one gut-healthy food a day. See what happens to your body and hanger level when you add gut-friendly ingredients, such as fermented foods that are naturally high in probiotics: sauerkraut, tempeh, and kimchi. All of these foods can help get the good bacteria we need back into the gut. And that can help our mood. For example, in a study in *Psychiatry Research,* 700 undergraduates were asked about their consumption of foods such as sauerkraut, kimchi, kombucha, yogurt, fermented soy products, pickles, and kefir.[21] They were also assessed for social anxiety. The outcome: students who ate fermented foods felt less social anxiety.

And that's not the only example. A 2013 UCLA study found that women who consumed yogurt twice a day for four weeks had lower levels of activity in the brain associated with mood and pain.[22] Also, researchers at the University of Virginia School of Medicine have reversed depression symptoms in mice by feeding them Lactobacillus, a probiotic bacteria found in yogurt containing live cultures.[23] These studies suggest promising ways to help people to feel less blue.

It's clear that there's a connection between probiotics and mood, and the right supplements can help you restore your gut bacteria and hopefully help you feel less anxious, which in turn can lead to less emotional eating. Also, probiotics help to manage how your body processes food. If you go this route, talk to your doctor about adding a probiotic to your diet to help restore and replenish many of the good bacteria that you need to help regulate your hunger and mood.

HUNGER HIJACKER #4: KICK THE HABIT

"Every day at ten o'clock I eat pretzels at my desk. I realized one day when I was out of my office at ten how routine this had become. I was annoyed that I didn't get my pretzels. I wasn't particularly hungry. But I missed the whole routine of it."

When it comes to my eating habits...

a) I'm very spontaneous about the way I eat.
b) I have a few habits around food.
c) I eat pretty much the same thing each day, in the same place.
d) I have very routine habits that I do every day.

"I have a really annoying habit when it comes to eating," Celeste divulged in my office. "Whenever I work at my desk, I go the kitchen first, get a snack, and then place it right next to my computer. I put it on the right-hand side of my screen. It's often a bag of something—chips, crackers, or popcorn. I eat while I work or distract myself on social media. It's like I can't even be at my computer without a snack."

I applauded Celeste for this awareness. A lot of habits are so routine that they become completely invisible to us. Then I asked Celeste not to change the habit, just to observe it.

The next time she had the snack at her desk, she immediately became annoyed with herself. The habit was painfully obvious. So, on her own, she decided not to stop snacking but to move the snack bag to the left-hand side of her computer.

"It was so interesting," she said. "I still brought the snack. But having to reach across the computer interrupted everything. When the bag was on the right, my hand unconsciously reached for the snacks. The result was that I was nibbling constantly. I realized right away when I moved it to the other side that it broke me out of this eating trance. I had to think about reaching across the computer to get a snack. It completely made me see this habit in a new way."

A habit is simply a behavior we do on repeat. Little to no thought is needed. They're things we do that aren't driven by emotions. And in the case of eating, habits are behaviors we have that aren't driven by hunger.

One of the first things my clients and I do is to take a really close look at the habits in their daily lives that might be at the root of feeling hangry or regretfull.

One of my clients talked about her "snooze habit." Every morning, when her alarm went off, she smacked the snooze button—sometimes more often than once. But this habit was definitely related to her being hangry. "If I just didn't hit snooze," she said, "I'd get up five minutes earlier. Then I'd have time to think through breakfast, instead of running out the door right from my shower and be starving by the time I got to work."

On the flip side, habits can be our best friend. Every night, like clockwork, I set my coffee pot to go off and be ready and waiting when I get up. It takes a step out of my morning. It's a choice I don't have to make. And it frees me up to make other choices—like what I'll eat to start the day.

The key is for us to choose our habits, rather than slipping into the same ones over and over again even when they're not serving us well. And when we do that, we can develop mindful habits that eliminate hanger.

One of the easiest ways to get out of old mindless habits is to interrupt our pattern. An interesting study that I tell my clients about is one that happened when London (the public transportation system) workers went on strike for two days.[24] When the Tube reopened, researchers looked at over a million data points taken from swipe cards to see what happened. Five percent of the commuters developed a new, more efficient route to use and stuck with it. Simply preventing them briefly from following a daily habit opened up their minds to forming a new one.

And here's how one of my clients, Melanie, reset her own

habits with the interruption technique. She would wander into the kitchen and mindlessly munch at night when she took her dogs out. Then one night, she put her dog gate in front of the kitchen door, so she couldn't mindlessly enter the kitchen. This new gate made her pause and think. And it helped her build a new habit.

Hangry to Happy

Nip habits in the bud! N—Notice habits. I—Interrupt habits. P—Position habits.

Notice habits: Notice, don't change your habits—at first. Make a list of three habits that may be contributing to your hanger. Your job is to pick just one habit, such as grazing on food when bored or snacking at night. Give it all of your attention, but just observe it. Notice everything about it. My clients are often surprised that I don't ask them to change it. But just observing your behavior often leads to change in itself. Think about your boss sitting in the room watching you work—what happens?

Interrupt habits: Habits are based on external cues that prompt you to do them. For example, when you see a bag of chips lying on the counter, you may automatically pick it up. So interrupt your habit. It might mean moving where you place your favorite snack or even getting rid of it. Maybe you start shopping at the back of the store instead of the front where you find your normal snacks. Or if you snack and watch TV, perhaps you sit in a different chair or room. Change up your routines. Ask yourself, "How can I interrupt my mindless eating habit?"

Position habits: Habits can get us in trouble. But they can also help. Too often we focus on trying to dislodge unhealthy habits when it is easier to build up mindful new ones. For instance: each night, place a snack bag next to your front door to pick up on your way out the next day. Or make it a habit to buy the same snack, like clockwork. Ask yourself right now, what habit would you like to ADD to your life, not take away? Most important, try "anchoring" the habit to another one that is already firmly in place. For example, maybe the first thing you do in the morning is make coffee. So you can begin to pack your lunch or snack as the coffee's brewing. With enough pairings of coffee with packing a lunch, these two habits will become linked. And it'll no longer be a struggle to make them happen.

HUNGER HIJACKER #5: NO TIME LIKE THE PRESENT

"Who has time for lunch? Not me—I've got more important things to do. Sitting down seems like such a waste of time when I've got a gazillion things to do. Sometimes I wish I had the time for a lunch break. It seems like a luxury."

If I skip a meal, it's usually because . . .

a) I'm too busy. I don't have time.
b) I'm trying to lose (or maintain) weight, so I avoid eating.
c) I forget because I have so much on my mind.
d) I rarely skip a meal.

The doctors and health care providers I've worked with for the past decade work extremely hard. They're on the go all day long. And sometimes that means missed meals.

I have one friend who never takes a lunch break. She prides herself on being "too busy" to stop to eat. She's a dedicated, in-demand doctor. Her waiting room's overflowing with clients. And her work schedule is hectic beyond belief most days. Perhaps more important, she wants to be efficient so she can get home to her family at a reasonable hour.

But by mid-afternoon, her staff starts to steer clear of her. That's because by 2:00 or 3:00, a pattern emerges. Her tone grows sharp. Her patience wears thin. I've even seen people duck into exam rooms or run into a different hallway just to avoid interacting with her.

It's possible she's simply tired. But as a psychologist, I believe hanger is rearing its ugly head, causing my friend to lose her typical level of compassion and kindness. And I'm not alone. I've heard more than one person joke that she needs someone to slip some chocolate or peanut butter into her coffee.

And if I were one of her patients, I'd rather wait a few minutes while she took the time she needs for lunch if that meant I could count on a consistently kind, friendly doctor whose patience and blood-sugar levels are regulated.

Research confirms the importance of making time to eat. However, nearly one quarter of individuals in the United States skip breakfast daily.[25] In a study of medical students, those who skipped breakfast had higher levels of fatigue and poor attention during clinical sessions.[26] I don't know about you, but I don't want a doctor walking into *my* exam room while suffering from fatigue and a lack of focus.

And it's not just doctors who are affected by skipping a meal. Consider the consequences when the person at the bank who is counting your money is overly hungry and can't concentrate. Or the mother next door who is babysitting your child. What about your child's bus driver or the accountant preparing your taxes? No matter what job we do in life, we need to remain sharp to be at our best.

It takes too much time or effort. Forgetting to eat. Not prioritizing meals. Trying to restrict calories. The reasons we give ourselves for skipping meals are never good ones. And skipping meals for any reason is always a recipe for hanger, fatigue, and flat energy.

There are often very distinct patterns to the way that people miss meals. For many, it's mornings. For others, it's lunchtime, because they are too busy and plow right through their lunch break. It might be evening, when you are rushing around dropping kids off at practices.

Be mindful of what stands in the way of a meal. Take note, when you miss a meal: how do you feel? Does it affect you physically? Do you find yourself dealing with low energy or motivation? Does it affect you emotionally? Do you feel more irritable? Or do you feel cognitive effects: all you can do is think about food, because your brain won't let you think about anything else besides what you can find in your fridge?

The good news is that your habits can be changed. They are not set in stone. Even a small meal or snack can snap us out of hanger.

Hangry to Happy

Change your mindset. Sometimes people skip meals because they feel that they must have a proper meal. But something is often better than nothing. So if all you can muster is sitting down for two minutes and mindfully eating a banana, your mood will likely thank you.

Think portable. If you typically eat breakfast, lunch, or dinner at work, consider packing portable foods and snacks. This includes easy-to-transport items and what I call "sturdy foods" such as granola bars, nuts, bananas, apples, cheese, and yogurt cups, which you can throw in a bag. Even if you are on the road during the day without access to a refrigerator, you can keep a small cooler with ice packs in your car for items that need to remain cold.

Overprepare. When making meatballs, you can just as easily prepare a dozen meatballs as you can six. Then you can freeze the unused portion and save it for days when you're extra-busy. It's much easier to stick with your plan when you already have premade meals—and all you need to do is defrost and reheat!

Subscription boxes. Although a more expensive option, if you just can't get to the grocery store, there are a host of cooking subscription clubs that will help you out! For a fee, these companies send all the ingredients and recipes for a home-cooked meal right to your door. If you are crunched for time, this may be an option to consider. Perhaps you reserve this alternative only for stressful times. Or maybe you set up an exchange with a friend. One week, you shop for two families. Create a box with all the items for a meal, including the ingredients and a recipe. Then, the next week your friend returns the favor.

HUNGER HIJACKER #6: DITCH THE DIET

"My friend calls me a professional dieter. I know everything there is to know about calories, portions, fat grams, etc. When I am not currently on a diet, I am anticipating my next fad diet. I hop from diet to diet. I know so much about food, but I don't know why it never seems to work for me. I end up starving and then eating like a lunatic."

When it comes to dieting . . .

a) I am always dieting.
b) I try to skip meals as often as possible.
c) I am sometimes on a diet.
d) I don't diet. I try to just eat mindfully.

Does this sound familiar?

Many of my clients try to restrict calories or go on diets as a way to manage their weight and hunger. They try the "I'll overpower my hunger" approach. They know they can't stop their hunger. So they decide they'll ignore it. It reminds me of a little kid who covers their ears and yells, "I don't hear you!"

Skipping a meal might make you feel like you are doing yourself a favor by cutting down on calories. But one of my first tasks with many of my clients is to convince them to stop fad dieting — right now.

When I tell them this, they look at me in horror.

"If I don't diet," they say, "then WHAT?"

So I review the evidence that proves dieting wreaks havoc on your body. Put simply, our bodies like consistency. When we diet, our body starts to work against us, trying to keep things consistent by maintaining the status quo.

A study at the Imperial College in London began by scanning the brains of volunteers to see what they looked like when they had eaten breakfast, and what their brains looked like when they had not. Then researchers asked subjects to go out and eat as much as they wanted. The result? Volunteers who skipped breakfast ate 250 calories more at their next meal. And volunteers who skipped breakfast also found high-calorie foods more tempting, particularly chocolate.[27]

In part, this is basic human psychology. We want what we can't have. But it's also biology. When you skip a meal, your gut releases hormones that send a message to the orbital frontal cortex. And this primes your brain to direct your thoughts toward tasty foods.

Restricting our calories at one meal just doesn't work — because it only makes us hungrier and more vulnerable to unhealthy decisions at the next meal. Not to mention that hanger is soon to follow.

My clients are pretty aware of how their mood changes when they are dieting. My client said, "My husband knows when I start a new diet. He says I am very edgy, and it's like walking on eggshells around me. He repeatedly asks me to stop because he doesn't like the evil twin dieting version of me."

Hangry to Happy

Lose the diet mentality. We often think thin = happy. But eating well is what truly leads to a positive mood. Instead of thinking about what you're taking off your plate, start to focus on what you put *on* it. The goal isn't restricting calories. It's about mindfully putting together a plate of nourishing, tasty food. In a study on happiness and college students, students who ate breakfast every day, ate more than eight servings of fruit and vegetables daily, and ate three meals in addition to one or two snacks per day had the highest happiness score.[28]

Shift your language. For a week, stop the diet-focused language—talking about or focusing on calories or portions. Instead, start asking yourself, "Am I eating mindfully?" A study published in the journal *Pediatrics* in 2018 showed that young adults whose parents had encouraged them to diet as teens were more likely to be overweight or obese; engage in dieting, binge eating, and unhealthy weight-control behaviors; and have lower body satisfaction when they became adults. And these disordered eating habits were still present fifteen years later! The researchers' recommendation: families should steer the conversation away from "dieting."[29]

Repeat this mantra. Important reminder: this is NOT a diet book. It's about honoring and understanding your hunger.

So whenever and whatever you choose to eat, repeat this mantra: *It's okay to eat mindfully.*

HUNGER HIJACKER #7: SWEETER THAN SUGAR

"My grandmother would remind me how even as a kid I used to dig through the stash of candy in her candy bowl on her coffee table. I've loved sugar for years and have a lot of daily cravings. Sometimes I only want something sweet. I have been known to get up at night, get dressed, and drive to the store to get some chocolate."

I would describe the role of sugar in my life like this . . .

a) I'm basically addicted to sugar.
b) Sugar is a main staple of my diet. I have a major sweet tooth!
c) I typically enjoy something sweet after a meal. I love eating a small piece of chocolate or a bite of cake after dinner.
d) A little bit of sugar goes a long way. I use it very sparingly and rather infrequently.
e) I prefer salty over sweet any day of the week.

My clients talk about all kinds of food: chocolate, comfort foods, mac and cheese, pizza. But there is one substance, hands down, that my clients struggle with the most: sugar.

Sugar is one of the only foods that my clients routinely pair with the words *addiction* and *craving*.

We all enjoy sugar—we are biologically wired to like it— but often my clients struggle with the role it plays in their lives and how it affects their moods. Even if you don't struggle with sugar overconsumption, eating sugar has immediate effects on your mood due to its impact on your glucose level, as we discussed in chapter one.

I've learned that sugar affects emotions in all kinds of ways. Some are positive. I think about the smile that comes across the face of my kids when they see I've made chocolate-chip cookies. Small amounts as treats often make us happy.

But eating large amounts of sugar and eating it when you are hungry have been connected to significant effects on mood that aren't as positive. Higher levels of sugar intake are linked with higher levels of depression.[30] But the direction of the correlation is not clear. Do people who are depressed eat more sugar, or does too much sugar lead to depression?

My clients often reach for sugar as a quick fix as hanger begins to set in — for good reason. Sugar works — temporarily. It's a sudden boost to blood glucose. And digging into a bag of M&M's is quick and easy. There is momentary relief from feeling hungry and irritable.

But what I find is that many of my clients get into a really difficult sugar cycle. When we look at their diet, sugar is a huge percentage of what they are eating. They are virtually surviving on it.

The cycle goes like this:

hungry: blood sugar is low
hanger sets in
grab some sugar
blood sugar rises quickly
temporary relief
crash
overly hungry — even more than before
repeat

Some of my clients are all too aware of this cycle. They know how much sugar they're eating, from the donut at breakfast to the candy bar in the afternoon. Others aren't as aware of the impact of sugar in their lives, because sugar is hidden everywhere, in less obvious places than donuts and candy bars. It's in everything from peanut butter to ketchup to salad dressing to "healthy" breakfast cereals.

Again, sugar is not "bad." But what's sweeter than sugar is when we are mindful of how sugar affects our moods and our bodies.

Hangry to Happy

Mind the sugar. Take a mindful look at the role and level of sugar intake you have in your life. Is it at the root of your hunger? Does it exacerbate it? Keep track of how sugar affects your mood and body. Whenever you eat something with added sugar, take note of your mood afterward. How does it affect your mood when you eat sugar as a treat—like a dessert after a meal? How is your mood different when you eat sugar in place of real food or fruit—reaching for a candy bar instead of a snack?

Take a brisk walk. Hungry? Try taking a walk! In a study on sugar cravings, participants who took a fifteen-minute brisk walk instead of eating sugar reported lower sugar cravings.[31]

Pause the sugar. Whenever you're about to reach for sugar, pause. Take a moment to identify where you are in the hanger cycle. Are you reaching for sugar because you are hangry, or about to be? Or is sugar being used as a treat? If it's a treat, no problem! But if you feel yourself spiraling into the hanger cycle, take a break—and mindfully feed your hunger. A helpful motto is "Feed hunger substance, not sugar."

Feel better with fruit. Try mindfully eating a piece of fruit, which can break the blood-sugar hanger cycle. Fruits do contain sugar, but they are also filled with fiber and nutrients. This helps you to digest fruit more slowly than sugary snack foods. And slower digestion helps regulate your hanger. Fruit can also improve your mood. In a study on sugar intake, including 70,000 women, researchers found higher chances of depression in those with a high intake of added and processed sugar but not in those with a high intake of naturally occurring sugars, such as those found in fruit.[32]

Skip artificial sweeteners. Zero-calorie sweeteners seem like they could be a saving grace. Many people assume that a no-calorie sweetener is better than regular sugar. Unfortunately, these synthetic sweeteners can make the problem worse, because artificial sweeteners confuse the signals in your brain and make you crave much higher levels of sweetness.

HUNGER HIJACKER #8: EAT REAL FOOD FOR YOUR MOOD

"I never thought much about eating foods that come out of a box and bag. But recently I've pondered how do some of these foods have such a long shelf life? Some packaged and sealed baked goods can last for ten years and never go bad—? And I am putting that in my body! When I started to pay attention, deep down I know that my body just feels gross after eating too much of it. And sometimes, I can even taste some of the chemicals in it that are likely used to preserve it."

What are your favorite processed snack foods? Select all that apply:

a) anything sweet, such as cookies, candy, and chocolate
b) salty foods, such as chips and french fries

c) pastries and donuts

d) other processed foods not on this list

e) none of the above: I don't snack and/or don't eat processed foods.

Can you get away with murder because you ate a Twinkie?

The "Twinkie defense" is an actual term, coined during the 1978 trial of Dan White, who was charged with the murder of Harvey Milk in San Francisco. White's psychiatrist indicated that his client had eaten a large quantity of sugary treats prior to the crime. He suggested that those sweets, coupled with White's depression, were a contributing factor in his loss of control.

In real life, the Twinkie defense was never a serious part of the Milk murder trial. But the idea gained traction in the popular mind, probably because all of us have lived through a version of it ourselves. Now, when we use the "Twinkie defense," what we really mean is: "I'm so sorry I was so grumpy. I had this amazing chocolate brownie cheesecake at lunch, but I ate way too much of it—and now I'm kind of snapping at people. Please forgive me." Or: "I ate something bad for me, and now I feel like crap. I don't even feel like myself!" Of course, for the majority of us, eating a snack isn't going to lead to murder. But eating highly processed food *can* lead to feelings of discomfort and agitation—and a poor mental state.

Some may argue that those first few bites of potato chips, chicken nuggets, packaged cookies, and sugary cereals are absolutely heavenly. They are! And if you're ravenously hungry, you may feel sure that those foods will provide you with the satisfaction you crave. But that satisfaction rarely lasts. Processed foods don't just wreak havoc with your blood-sugar levels. They often don't truly satisfy hunger.

Have you ever felt hungry, even shortly after eating? Most likely, what you ate did nothing for your body, nutritionally speaking. And nothing leaves you hungrier than processed foods, including zero-calorie sweeteners that give you literally nothing and leave you wanting more.

And junk food can affect your mood, too. According to a study from the University of California at San Diego's School of Medicine, too much junk can actually make you mean! In a study of the diets and behaviors of nearly 1,000 men and women, researchers found that a higher intake of trans fat was significantly tied to an increase in aggression and irritability.[33]

One of the major aha! moments my clients have in the Hanger Management program is when they start to track what happens to their bodies when they eat an abundance of processed foods. They begin to recognize that some foods make them feel good, some don't do much but satiate hunger, and some foods simply don't sit well with the body. Once they know that, they can make more mindful decisions.

A client of mine told me a story about cinnamon rolls. She was at the airport and picked up the sweet smell of cinnamon rolls. The next thing she knew, she was following the scent as if she was being led by the pied piper. She was mesmerized by the smell, but then she had a brief moment of pause.

"These are not my mom's cinnamon rolls," she reminded herself. "They're from an airport vendor." But as the smell lured her in, she quickly dismissed that thought. Minutes later, she had quickly eaten a humongous cinnamon roll about the size of a salad plate, and was licking icing off her fingers.

Remembering our talks, she didn't judge herself. Instead, she just noticed her reaction. What struck her most was her disappointment. The roll she'd eaten was not baked completely, so it was damp in the middle, but she had eaten it anyway. It completely lacked the wonderful consistency of the rolls her mother made. And she said it felt like a rock in her stomach for the next few hours. When we talked next, she told me that remembering how the experience affected her body and mood was the biggest deterrent for the next time she smelled the glorious scent of cinnamon rolls in an airport.

Hangry to Happy

Know what you're dealing with. First, it's important to identify the processed foods in your life. Sometimes they are tough to spot! Foods that are fried, baked, frozen, canned, or packaged are suspect. Step one is simple: read the labels. Just turn it over and see what's inside. Is the paragraph of ingredients short, medium, or long? You don't need to become an expert on every ingredient. Just be mindful of what is in your food.

Do a post-bite huddle. No matter what kind of food you eat, whether processed or not, take a moment to mindfully huddle up and note the immediate impact. Once it is down the hatch, check in with these three S's. How does it **S**it in your stomach, how does it **S**atisfy you, and how does it **S**hift your feelings?

Test it out. Experiment with different ways to prepare food. Notice how they taste to you and how different kinds of preparation influence your mood. Sometimes the way a food is prepared even affects your level of satisfaction, or satiety. For example, a study on apples showed that people felt fuller when they ate a whole apple, as opposed to drinking apple juice or eating applesauce before a meal. Do you feel the same?[34]

Get the real deal. One way to cut down on processed foods is to buy local. For example, small bakeries don't usually fill their bread with preservatives the way big bread companies do in order to keep them on shelves for long periods of time. Or learn how to cook your favorite processed foods yourself. As Michael Pollan advises, if you love fries, that's great—just make them yourself.

HUNGER HIJACKER #9: IN HOT WATER

"Water is just so boring. I don't drink nearly enough in a day—I can tell because my pee is a bright yellow color."

I get thirsty...

a) all the time, because I forget to drink water.
b) sometimes. I rarely drink water unless it is served to me at a restaurant.
c) rarely. I make an active effort to drink more water but don't hit the mark every day.
d) almost never because I drink a lot of water.

Hanger isn't just about lack of food.

Not getting enough water can make us vulnerable to hanger, too.

One of my clients tells a story about hiking in the woods with her family. They came prepared with backpacks, snacks, etc. But they forgot to bring the most important thing—water. They had only one little bottle to share among three of them.

As the day proceeded, it got hot and tempers got short. They began to fight over tiny sips of water from the water bottle and who had gotten more.

They had food. Snacks helped a bit—but the thirst led to edgy moods and lethargy.

Research has shown that dehydration, even small amounts of it, negatively affects your mood and thinking. And lack of water leads to fatigue and lack of mental alertness. It can even lead to death!

Think of a time when you noticed that you were running low on water. Maybe it was working outside on the lawn. Or perhaps you drank a lot of coffee—but didn't drink any water in the morning. Do you remember feeling thirsty—and irritable? This bad mood comes from some of the same mechanisms that cause hanger.

The good news is that when you do hydrate, water improves your mood and ability to think clearly almost immediately. In a recent study, children and adult participants were offered either no water, 25 milliliters, or 300 milliliters to drink.[35] Researchers tested participant performance before drinking water and twenty minutes after drinking or after going without a drink.

For both children and adults, a large drink (300 ml) was necessary to reduce thirst. But even a small drink (25 ml) was sufficient to improve visual attention. Both children and adults had better visual attention even when they drank small amounts of fluid. In adults, a large drink also improved digit span—how long a string of numbers they could recall. Participants who were thirsty, on the other hand, performed poorly on a memory task.

Another study observed the relationship between a habit of drinking water and mood.[36] One hundred twenty healthy women recorded all the food and fluids they consumed for five consecutive days. Participants completed assessments on their level of tension, depression, anger, vigor, confusion, and mood. The interesting finding: researchers learned they could predict a subject's mood just by looking at how much water she'd been drinking!

Ever wished you had a magic potion to drink that could

improve your memory and your mood? You do—and it's as close by as the kitchen sink or the office water cooler.

Hangry to Happy

To prevent thirst-induced moodiness and to improve mental sharpness—which gives you an advantage when you are making food choices—getting enough water is key.

Tune in. Be mindful of signs that you are running low on water. Your body gives you some distinct clues. Which signs apply to you? The goal is to hydrate well to *prevent* these cues from popping up.

- **Unusual Hunger.** Thirst and appetite are both regulated by the hypothalamus. The signals between these two functions can get crossed and make you think you are hungry when you are really thirsty. *If you tend to run low on water, pause when your mind says, "I'm hungry" and assess whether you need water or food.*
- **Fatigue or Exhaustion.** Exhaustion happens when lactic acid builds up and glucose production shuts down.
- **Constipation.** Hydration helps your system digest and eliminate food well.
- **Bad Breath.** There is not enough saliva to clean out your mouth when you are dehydrated. A dry mouth leads to bad breath.
- **Dark Urine**. The darker the color, the more dehydrated you are. In general, the lighter your pee, the better (but nearly clear is a sign of over-hydration).
- **Headaches.** Lack of water makes your brain tissue shrink and pull away from your skull, setting off pain receptors.
- **No Tears.** Dry eyes mean your mucous membranes don't have enough water.

- **Overheating.** Fluids help regulate your body temperature.
- **Muscle Cramping.** To contract efficiently, muscles need sodium and potassium in water.
- **Lightheadedness.** When you are dehydrated, your blood fluid levels drop, lowering your blood pressure and reducing circulation to the brain.

Try the 3-second pinch. Gently pinch the skin on the back of your hand or arm and pull up about one centimeter before letting go. If the skin stays raised for a moment and then slowly returns to normal, this could be a sign of dehydration. This is called the turgor test. It is a quick way to tell if you are running low on water. Your skin loses elasticity when it lacks water, so it doesn't return to its normal shape as quickly as usual. Ideally it should spring back to its original position immediately.

Be mindful of thirst vampires. Some foods and drinks suck the hydration right out of you! Caffeinated coffee, soda, and energy drinks all undo your efforts to stay hydrated. They are diuretics, meaning they cause you to produce urine and pee more frequently. And excessive salt can cause the body to pull water from your cells to maintain healthy sodium levels in the blood. Make sure to counter every thirst vampire with more hydration.

Mindfully hydrate. If you find yourself chronically low on water and you believe this may be increasing your appetite and hanger level, turn to Tip #32.

SUMMARY OF HANGRY HIJACKERS

Now you know some of the factors that can hijack your hunger: things that can grab you in the middle of an otherwise good day and drag you down a mindless eating path. Remember, these factors don't make it impossible to eat mindfully. But they make it a lot more challenging.

Before you leave this chapter, make a check next to the factors that have the most impact on you. You may even want to rank on a scale from 1 to 10 how much you suspect each of these factors affects how you eat. You'll notice some aren't an issue. Maybe you get solid sleep, no problem. But perhaps you paused when it came to sugar and said, "Yep, that's me!"

____ my stress level
____ the amount of sleep I get
____ what is happening in my gut
____ my habits
____ skipping meals
____ dieting or trying to restrict calories
____ eating lots of sugar/sweets
____ eating a lot of processed food
____ not drinking enough water

What did you check? Whatever resonated the most with you, that's a great place to start. And after you've addressed the hunger hijackers in your life, you'll find mindful eating much easier and enjoyable!

Hanger-Free Homes and Hangouts

Where do you get the hangriest?

At home?

At the office?

On vacation?

In your car?

This is one of my first questions to my clients. What I find is that it's likely that there are some locations where hanger is a daily occurrence and other places where hanger never even enters the picture.

The places where hanger is quick to arise are like quicksand for mindful eating. You step into the environment and wham! You sink. Even if you walk in with the best intentions, they sometimes fly out the window when your hanger triggers are present.

Sometimes environments encourage mindless eating—they make food easy to grab without any thought. For example, my friend used to keep a bowl of mixed nuts on her counter. I can't tell you the number of times I have witnessed people at her house, standing around chatting, dipping into this nut bowl, popping one or two in and then a handful, not because they were hungry, but because it was just there, within reach.

On the flip side, it's possible to arrange your surroundings to make your food choices more deliberate and conscious. Granted, you can't always control your environment. For example, my office is right next to a donut shop. (No joke!) There is nothing I can do about that. But in places where you can make a mindful environment, why not give yourself a head start on mindful eating?

In the Hanger Management program, we learn how to tune in to the *internal* hunger cues that trigger us to eat. Some of the signs that we need to eat are clear cut, like a loud, rumbly belly. Others are more subtle, like low energy. But what studies show is that we often eat in response not to our internal cues but to cues *outside* ourselves. For example: you see a commercial for pizza. You weren't hungry for pizza two minutes ago. But now, bubbly cheese and thick crust is all you can think about.

The Hanger Management program is about strengthening your ability to hear your internal hunger no matter where you find yourself—and to spot when you are just going with the flow, like diving into buffalo chicken wings and dip at retirement party just because others around you are snacking on it.

So take a mindful look around you. You might start with your car, your kitchen, your bedroom, or your closet. Wherever it is, start to notice how your surroundings shape your food choices.

HANGER FREE #10: STEP UP TO THE PLATE

"Food is not just eating energy. It's an experience." — *Guy Fieri*

When I eat, I eat off of...

a) right out of the fast-food bag.
b) a napkin.

c) a paper plate.

d) everyday dishes.

e) very nice dishes, such as pretty china.

My mother loves nice dishes. She has a set of china from her mother and other sets inherited from other relatives. For her, eating has always been an experience. At the holidays, the big question is always which dishes to use. The holiday-themed dishes? The bone-colored plates with gold rims that she inherited from her mother? The ones from my aunt, with their rose pattern? The backdrop that her food is served on matters to her.

One of the most important things she taught me about dishes is to use them. Often, people save their "good" dishes for presenting food well for a special occasion. But to my mom, beautiful dishes were never just for holidays or fancy dinners. "What are we saving them for," she'd joke, "a visit from the queen?" Then she'd laugh and set the table.

To her, her family was special enough for setting a pretty table all the time. We didn't always use the fancy ones, but she regularly made sure the table looked nice. She cleared off the clutter—homework, books, toys, or mail. Then she made sure everyone had a plate, silverware, a glass, and a napkin. We did not eat out of a fast-food bag at the table.

What research says, time and again, is that the way food looks matters to all of us. In fact, it matters so much that the way food looks influences how good it tastes to us. That's why restaurants go through a great deal of effort to create table ambience and plate the food in an attractive manner. They know it's all part of the experience of eating.

Most of my clients tell me that they spend very little time thinking about the way their food is served. When they're hangry, they eat right out of the french-fry bag, snack right out of the cereal box, take ham right out of the deli bag and pop it into their mouth. If you are doing these things, it may be a sign that you really struggle with hanger.

The good news is that, with just a little thought, you can make a big impact on how much you enjoy your food. The way we plate food has an impact on our appetite, how much we like a dish, what we're willing to purchase, and even how full we feel. And we can affect all these things without drastically changing what we eat and without extra cost, just by paying a little attention to the visual experience of a snack or meal.[37]

Hangry to Happy

Portion perception. A study in the journal *Appetite* examined how food placement affects perception of the portion.[38] The punchline: when food is spread out on a plate, it looks like more to us than when it's served in a stack. And food placed right in the middle of a plate seems like a larger portion than the same amount pushed over to the side. So help your brain feel like you're getting more, by spreading your food over your plate, starting in the middle.

Bright plates. Studies show that the color of plates changes your perception of how food tastes.[39] We all want that! People tend to perceive food as more flavorful—sweeter and saltier—when served on plates in bright colors, such as red, blue, yellow, and green. Using red plates (which you will learn more about in a later tip) has multiple benefits!

Watch the edge. People tend to feel like they have more food on their plate when the plate has a colored rim around the edge, due to a phenomenon called the Delboeuf illusion.[40] Picture two identical shaded circles. One has a tight circle around it, like the rim around a plate. The surrounding circle makes what is inside look larger, so it seems as if there is more food on the plate. We feel more satisfied when we have the perception that we are eating more. So help yourself to feel more satisfied by using dishes with a colored rim around the edge!

Plates with messages. Plates don't have to be boring. I have plates that give helpful reminders like "Eat mindfully," "Savor," and "Enjoy." Even when I'm distracted or in a rush, they help me stay on track. You can even create a mindful placemat with positive messages or download a free one from my website, www .eatingmindfully.com.

HANGER FREE #11: OUT OF SIGHT, OUT OF MIND

"I struggle with what I call "fly-by eating." I breeze through the kitchen door, stick my hand in an open bag of cheese curls, and walk out with my handful. Then I get mad at myself. I didn't really need, want, or enjoy it at all. I was just passing by and grabbed snacks without even thinking."

When food is around,

a) I will grab a bite totally without thinking.
b) I want it, regardless of whether or not I'm hungry.
c) I eat only if I am hungry but am not picky about my options if I am.
d) I think through my hunger level and whether I want to eat a particular food or not.

Does this sound familiar? One minute you're working at your desk. The next, your hand is in a glass jar of chocolate kisses, and there's a growing pile of wrappers next to your computer.

"Holy cow," you think. "How did I eat all of those?"

Not only that, but all that chocolate didn't alleviate your hunger. And it didn't give you much pleasure, either. In fact, you barely remember eating it. You ate it just *because it was there.*

Where we place things matters. We put bedrooms in the backs of our houses to avoid street noise. We put cosmetics behind bathroom mirrors so they're out of sight but just where we need them. We put the remote near our couch so we don't have to get up to find it.

Where we put our food matters, too.

The psychological *proximity principle* states that the closer we are to food, the more likely we are to eat it. Don't get me wrong. Eating is not a bad thing. But eating mindlessly, without thinking about it, can lead to feeling hangry and regretfull. My clients hate when they eat something mindlessly. It doesn't fill them up, and they don't enjoy it.

One of my clients realized that her freezer was a big source of mindless eating. Whenever she opened it to pull out something healthy to make for dinner, the first thing she spied was a pint of ice cream. She wasn't thinking about ice cream. She wasn't even hungry. But before she knew it, the ice cream was in her hand, and she was eating spoonfuls directly from the container. It irritated her. She didn't want to stop eating ice cream altogether, but she didn't want to eat it mindlessly before dinner.

The solution we came up with together wasn't rocket science, but it worked. She just moved the ice cream to the back of the freezer. When she opened the door, it wasn't the first thing she saw. Getting the ice cream out required moving frozen soup, a package of beef, and popsicles. And that cut down on the "it's right there" trap.

The research seems to agree with her intervention as well. In

one study, researchers put bowls of chocolate in front of participants.[41] The bowls were either 70 centimeters away, or much
closer—only 20 centimeters. Those that sat closer to the chocolate, ate more—no surprise!

But it's not just chocolate that we eat when it's close at hand. In
another study, grapes, crackers, and chocolate were put at vary-
ing distances—either six feet away or within arm's reach.[42] The
researchers found that people not only ate chocolate when it was
closer, but they also filled up more on the healthier grapes and
crackers.

This is actually incredibly good news. One of the easiest
things you can do to cut down on mindless eating and increase
your chances of conscious eating is rearranging your environment.

It's human nature to reach for food that's close by. So don't be
hard on yourself if you do. Instead, hack the process. Build an
environment where it's harder to eat mindlessly and easier to eat
the good stuff that really gives you energy and fills you up.

Hangry to Happy

Out of sight, out of mind. Take a tour of your kitchen. Look
around. Is there anything on your counter that may contribute to
mindless eating? A bag of chips, a bottle of soda, a cookie jar, a
box? You don't have to throw it away. Just place it in a cupboard,
in a bag that you can't see through.

Within-reach principle. Sit at your desk and do a sweep
with your arm. Is there anything edible within reach? As the
study above suggests, move it at least 70 centimeters (a little over
two feet) away from you. Better yet, put it in a drawer instead.
This will significantly cut down on mindless snacking.

Mindful food placement. Use proximity to your advantage with healthy food. Pick something that does make you feel

good when you eat it and put it strategically nearby—on your desk, in a bowl on your counter, or anywhere you can see it.

HANGER FREE #12: A MINDFUL MAKEOVER

"Sometimes I feel like talking myself into eating good things is like trying to convince a fish to jump into water. I know what's healthy. It's such a struggle to actually do it."

About healthy foods:

a) I don't like healthy foods and struggle to eat them.
b) I like healthy foods but have trouble choosing them.
c) I like healthy foods and eat them some of the time.
d) I have healthy foods available and eat them all the time.

Anyone who comes to my office will tell you that they always see the same thing on my desk, every time: an apple.

I put it front and center on my monitor, so I can't avoid seeing it when I type my notes.

I eat apples all the time—in part, because I love them. But, also, I would much rather snack on an apple that is right in front of me than scrounge quarters from the bottom of my purse and walk down the hall to the vending machine. The trip to the vending machine doesn't just take money; it takes time. Choosing the apple is a no-brainer.

My clients generally like healthy foods. But some of them don't eat them as much as they'd like. "How do I choose an apple over chocolate?" they ask me. "I like my apples, but I love chocolate, too."

I understand the struggle to choose. In psychology, researchers have tried to help make mindful choices less of a struggle, through something called "choice architecture." Choice architecture is all about making small, low-cost changes in what food is convenient, attractive, and visible, with strategies like offering healthy items as default selections in grab-and-go combinations. It aims to make healthy food the easy option instead of the hard one.

For instance, one study looked at what happens when you move around salad bar options.[43] Over the course of two months, researchers simply varied the location of eight salad ingredients— broccoli, shredded cheese, chicken, cucumbers, hard-boiled eggs, mushrooms, olives, and tomatoes. What the researchers discovered was that people took more of the ingredients that were placed on the edges than the ones in the middle. According to the researcher's calculations, just moving around these items over a year's time could make a difference of half a pound in a person's weight.

This should make you pause for a moment, and do a double take about how we make our choices. It does for me. Are you choosing something because you like it? Or just because it is right in front of you?

And most important, how can you use that information to your advantage?

Studies show that you can make choices that change your behavior for the better without even having to think about it. For example, individuals drink more water while eating if the water pitcher is on the table, rather than 20 or 40 feet away.[44] In other words, you'll probably drink more water with a meal if water is sitting in front of you.

Other studies looked at what happens when food is moved from the back of the grocery store to the front.[45] Researchers found that when fruits and vegetables were moved into attractive displays near the front of the store, people bought more of them. It makes sense. How many times have you impulse-bought a soda, a candy bar, or mints as you wait in line to buy groceries, just because they're there?

Stores know we're going to reach for whatever food is convenient. And we can use that same principle to become our own food-choice architects at home and work. Think about how to make eating healthy food less of a struggle, even effortless. Then engineer your environment so it's hard *not* to eat healthy, mindful foods you love.

Hangry to Happy

Be your own choice architect. A banana in the hand is worth five in the grocery bag. So put food that you want to eat *in your sight*. Place healthy snacks out in the open. Make foods you want to eat very visible in clear containers or baggies. Even removing the lid on a nut jar can help you to choose them as a healthy snack more often. Take fruit out of the bag.

Desk snacks. Place a healthy snack right on your desk, so you can't ignore it. That way, you'll eat more of the good stuff and be less willing to mindlessly grab whatever else you see.

On-the-go snacks. Put a bowl of mindful snacks *right next* to your door, so you grab a snack on the way out without having to hunt for it at the last minute.

Pre-cut veggies. One of the best investments my clients talk about is buying cut-up vegetables—because when fruit or vegetables are already cut, the odds of our eating them go up. Pre-cut produce may cost a bit more, but think of it as an investment in your health. And if you eat them instead of letting them go bad, it's a double win. So think about where you place them in the fridge. If you put them in the crisper drawer, you can wave goodbye to them for good, as it's easy to completely forget about them there. Instead, place fruits and veggies in view in your refrigerator, not in a drawer.

Veggie hack. Buy frozen veggies, which are easy to pour into pasta and other dishes without the bother of prepping them.

Water on hand. As the study above highlighted, always put water on the table in a pitcher so you don't have to get up to refill. Keeping a water pitcher handy is one of the easiest things you can do to help yourself and your family manage hunger levels more mindfully. And carry a refillable water bottle with you daily. I keep an emergency case of water bottles in my car trunk in case I need one or someone else does.

Car snacks. Tuck some mindful snacks in the armrest or the side pockets of your car. This can help you to fill up on snacks that are right under your nose instead of mindlessly swinging through the fast-food drive-through.

HANGER FREE #13: WATCH HOW YOU WATCH

I keep telling myself, just one more episode and I will go to bed. But I get completely hooked and drawn in. Then I can't stop until I have watched the entire season. And I snack while I am watching. Sometimes I take a break between episodes and get a different snack.

When I binge-watch TV . . .

a) I snack the whole time.
b) I snack at least once.
c) I may stop the show when I'm hungry, get a snack, and get right back to it.
d) I don't snack at all.

During the decade I've been a psychologist, technology has changed a lot.

And so has the way it affects how we eat.

Sarah is a great example of someone who didn't have an issue with mindless eating—until the invention of on-demand TV. Many of us would agree that on-demand television is one of the best inventions ever! And in our session, Sarah said that binge-watching shows could be helpful when she needed to sit still to rest or relax. She's an on-the-go, slightly anxious mom who can find it hard to slow down. Becoming engrossed in a show has helped her to unwind.

The downside, for Sarah, and many others: sinking into a TV program is one of the biggest triggers of mindless eating.[46] Often, people who struggle with binge-watching TV also struggle with mindless eating and binge-eating. They both provide the same feeling—escape and pleasure. Put them together and you get the perfect hiatus from the world.

But the more we watch, studies show, the more we eat. And when we watch action-packed or sad content, we eat even more than when we watch other kinds of shows.

That was true for Sarah. When she was distracted and in a comfort zone, she tended to eat more. But in our work together, she started to be mindful of the situation and how it affected her habits. She realized that bingeable TV programs include subtle advertisements for food directly in the program, partly because people who binge programs often watch them without commercials. When she saw characters munching or images of tasty food, she was triggered to eat.

Watching TV series in the past didn't require us to self-regulate or tell ourselves "Enough!" Each series only had one episode a week. Period.

But now we need to use the front part of our brain, the prefrontal cortex. It makes executive decisions and tells us when to say "stop" or "more" to pleasure. When we're in a happy state, experiencing pleasure, our brains release dopamine, the neurotransmitter that flows when we enjoy anything that makes us feel good: sex, eating, or watching hours of good TV. It's like a "hit" to the brain. But you can get too much of a good thing and overdose on just about anything, including binge-watching TV. The result? We start to feel numb. Our brain wants more dopamine, so we continue the activity to get more. We might not be conscious of it, but that's what's happening in the brain.

Some of my clients also have another issue related to binge-watching: they stay up into the wee hours of the night to do it. This has a big impact on their health and hanger. Not only are they dragging the next day, but missing sleep skews your appetite hormones, as discussed in Tip #2 (Sleep Tight for a Mindful Appetite). Losing even one hour of sleep can make you feel hungrier. And when people lose sleep, they make more decisions they regret about food—and just about everything else in their lives.

So we need to practice putting on the brakes.

Hangry to Happy

Set mindful limits. Choose how many episodes, or how much time you want to spend, in advance. That will make it easier for you to make mindful decisions when the time comes to stop watching.

Skip commercials. If there are commercials, fast-forward past them so you don't see the pizza and chip ads, especially if you are someone who struggles with mindless eating or intense cravings!

Save sleep. Don't let what I call Binge Marathon Munching reduce your sleep. Go to bed at a reasonable time, to the best of your ability. Set a deadline. No watching past that time!

Use the buddy system. Watch with a buddy who will help keep you honest about your watching time. Bonus: we tend to eat less when we have an audience.

Go cold turkey. One strong option: just don't eat and watch TV at the same time. Period. Make it a goal to turn off the TV if you have a snack, or move to a table instead of the couch. Give eating your full attention.

Avoid alcohol. Try to avoid using alcohol or other substances while binge-watching TV. Substances make it even harder to stop watching and also increase the likelihood of mindless eating.

Ban the bag. If you do eat while watching, portion it out into a bowl or plate. Don't eat right out of the bag or box.

Keep your hands moving. One of my clients knits while she watches TV, and another client works on a project to keep her hands busy. It's impossible, she says, to snack and knit at the same time.

HANGER FREE #14: UNPLUG YOUR APPETITE

"I sit across from my husband at the kitchen table. But we are both looking at our phones, not talking to each other as we eat. Sometimes we even text each other from across the table at meals."

When I eat...

a) my nose is buried in the phone.
b) I check my phone any time I get an alert.
c) I turn off my phone and focus on what I am eating.

"My boyfriend just phubbed me!" my client said.

Phubbed was a new word for me. Like *hanger,* it's a slang combination of two words—in this case, *phone* and *snubbed*—mashed together, which describes one way technology affects your social relationships. And if it's ever happened to you, you probably felt like the person *phubbing* you was disrespectful or rude.

As far as I know, no one's invented a word yet to describe snubbing your *food* in favor of your phone. But often our phones grab our complete attention while we snack. We've got the snack in one hand, and with the other we're scrolling through our social media accounts.

The problem is that when we're buried in a phone while we eat snacks or meals, we don't enjoy our food as much, and we don't eat as mindfully.

A study in the journal of *Experimental Social Psychology* observed the impact of technology on the eating habits of three hundred participants.[47] Researchers sent them out to dinner, then investigated what happened as they ate. One group had their phones, and another group did not. The people who had their phones at the table used them for a whopping 11 percent of the meal—a little more than one minute out of every ten. People who used their phones while eating reported feeling more distracted and less socially engaged. They also mentioned a significant drop in the enjoyment of their meal.

If it's tough for you to put your phone aside during meals, you aren't alone. My clients often struggle with changing this habit. These days, our phones are glued to our hands. We use them for entertainment, companionship, and distraction.

A study of the eating habits of 2,000 Americans found that many of us are increasingly distracted when eating. About 29 percent of people say their phone now accompanies EVERY meal they eat. Over half of those studied say their phone is a mainstay at most of their meals. Only 17 percent say they never have their phone at the table.[48]

Do you think "Yikes! No way!" when you consider putting your phone aside? That's okay. Remember, it's just for a short period of time. And the benefits are huge. You'll enjoy your meal more. And you'll be much more conscious of what and how much you eat.

Hangry to Happy

Keep it off the table. Try a simple trick that doesn't involve changing your food at all! Leave your smartphone in the car or another room, not just in your bag or turned over on the table. A study in the *Journal of the Association for Consumer Research* found that a phone can still engage your mind even if it is on silent, powered off, or hidden.[49] If we see it, we think about it—who might be sending a message or what you might look up. And because it still demands your attention even if you aren't using it when you know it is near, the study found that the presence of a smartphone reduced people's working memory and problem-solving abilities.

Turn off the ringer. If you can't leave your phone outside the room, remember that sounds are a big distractor from meals and snacks. Even the ding of an email alert can break your focus. A study in the *Journal of Experimental Psychology* found that hearing your phone buzz or ring, even if you don't respond to it, can hurt your performance on cognitive tasks.[50] Suddenly you're wondering "Who can that be? What do they want?" You're no longer thinking of what you're eating or enjoying your food or company. At the table, phone silence is golden.

Use a tech drop box. Make going tech-free fun. Find a colorful box where everyone deposits their electronics before meals—including you. Ideally, it may be near an outlet for people to recharge. This gets everyone in the habit of not texting during meals.

Check in once in a while—mindfully. If you just can't step away from the phone, check it mindfully. As noted, people can become anxious when separated from their phones. And we don't make great food decisions when we are anxious. So checking our phones may sometimes reduce our anxiety and help us to think more clearly about what we eat. But often, we check our phones without really needing to. Many people do it without thinking, as an automatic habit. If you want to check your phone during mealtimes, do it consciously. Start the meal with a plan: "After I eat my sandwich, I'll take a break and look at my phone. Then I'll put my phone away and eat my apple." When you're not trying to eat and check your phone at the same time, you can do both things more mindfully.

HANGER FREE #15: AVOIDING SNACK-CIDENTS

"I have a lot of snack accidents throughout the day. Often, it's when I am waiting as dinner is cooking. I start to snack because I am so hungry. Then that snack turns into a lot of sampling and snacking when I had no intention of that happening. And I'm no longer hungry for the meal I was waiting for."

When it comes to snacking...

a) I snack a lot, and often too much.
b) Sometimes I start snacking and accidentally eat too much.
c) I never snack and eat only at designated times, even if it means I get hangry between meals.
d) I love to snack, and I am mindful of my portions.

"Snack-cidents" is what my clients call it when they unintentionally wind up eating more than they meant to as a snack.

It happens completely unintentionally. You reach for a handful of cashews, but before you know it, half the canister is gone. And it doesn't just take away your hunger. It makes you uncomfortably full.

It can happen anywhere. You might be standing in the kitchen when suddenly your hand is snaking into an open bag of chips on the counter. Or you might be at work, when out of the corner of your eye, you see a bowl of granola bars. Before you know it, you're surrounded by empty wrappers. You didn't mean for it to go down like this.

Snack-cidents sneak up on my clients most often at moments when they genuinely need a snack. They are moderately aware that they are hungry. But they get busy and sink into a mindless zone. And then they lose track of how much they're eating. When they're not paying attention, it's easy to go beyond their appetite. A few bites would have taken the edge off their hunger. But snacking snowballs.

The downside is that snack-cidents make some of my clients suspicious of having any snacks at all. They steer clear of snacks because they don't want to have a snack-cident. But then, when they're genuinely hungry, they don't know what to do.

Other clients of mine sometimes graze all day long. When I ask what they ate today, or how much, they throw up their hands and say, "I have no idea." They don't mean to overeat. But when they graze without thinking, it's too easy to do.

This isn't uncommon. One study on snacking looked at the impact of whether we label what we eat a snack or a meal—and if where we eat our snacks and meals makes a difference.[51] Eighty female participants were offered pasta. Some of it was labeled a snack and eaten from a container while standing. And some was described as a meal and eaten from a plate while seated at a table. Researchers found that people ate more when the pasta was labeled a snack and standing up than while eating it from a plate. It's no surprise. We often pay less attention to the amount we eat when we consider it to be "just a snack." And when we stand and eat, we get very distracted.

After the pasta, participants were offered chocolate. Those who thought they had just eaten a pasta snack ate more chocolate than those who had eaten what they thought of as a meal. The researchers suggest that those who thought they ate a snack likely ate more because they thought they would be hungry later— since all they'd had was "just a snack."

Hangry to Happy

I remind my Hanger Management clients that snacks are great— and necessary! Snacks help tremendously to manage hunger and ward off hanger. The key is to bring mindfulness to snacking. What we learn from this study is that if you are having a snack, it's important to choose the right snack.

Snack with intention. Use this little acronym to help you to avoid unintentional eating.

- **S**—Slow down. Consciously choose a snack. Don't just eat the first thing you see or can reach. Ask yourself what you really want.
- **N**—Notice your hunger. How hungry are you, on a scale from 1 (extremely empty) to 10 (completely full)? Given your rating, do you need a big or little snack?
- **A**—Ask yourself, what are my options? Name three possible snacks you could have right now.

C—Choose thoughtfully. Ask yourself, will this snack meet my needs? Will it take the edge off my hunger or give me a taste of what I really desire?

K—Kindness. As you snack, ask yourself, "Am I being kind to my body right now? Would it be mindful to stop or to keep eating?" If you want another bite, continue to eat until you are satisfied.

Set up snack cues. To help keep you in the mindset of a snack, take advice from the study mentioned above. Consciously think of the word *snack*. Use a small plate or ramekin instead of a dinner plate or salad bowl—items we use for meals. Or, try placing your snack on a napkin, which is a very clear reminder to stay in a snack mindset. Or label your baggie with the word *snack*. Then, have a seat!

HANGER FREE #16: "STOPLIGHT" EATING

"I love in the Hanger Management program that some of the tips are really easy and take very little effort. One of my favorite tips has been using a red plate. I went out and bought one immediately. At home, I always eat my snack off it. I remind myself that the point is not to avoid or skip the snack, but to slow down the pace. It's a subtle reminder—which I need because I have so much on my mind."

When it's time for me to stop eating...

a) I just eat until it's gone.
b) I consciously have to tell myself to stop eating once I feel full.
c) I create reminders to help me to remember to stop eating.

    d) I automatically stop eating when I'm full, without much effort or thought.

One of my clients did an experiment on food colors for her high school science fair recently. She looked at the impact of color on how people rate their food. Her test case was two white cakes: one dyed strawberry pink, and the other dark blue.

You probably won't be surprised by her results. Although the two cakes tasted exactly the same, the pink was rated as far tastier.

My client chose blue because blue isn't usually considered an appetizing color for food — except for blueberries. Some of that may be biological. Not many foods that occur in nature are blue. We're more accustomed to seeing red foods, like the pink color iron gives to meat, or green foods, from the chlorophyll in plants. A recent study even found that putting food under blue lights makes it less appetizing to men, and they eat less of it.[52, 53]

Marketers use color all the time to influence how much we like the taste of various foods. For example, the color of wine labels influences our expectations of how the wine inside will taste. Red and black labels are most likely to create tangy flavor expectations. But red and orange labels are most associated with fruity and flowery flavors.[54]

And color doesn't just influence how we expect food to taste. It changes our behavior.

And the color red is one of the most powerful colors — it affects both how we think and what we actually do. Think about a stop sign. Even if you saw it without the words, you would still stop. You're reacting to the color.

And it's been proven to work in how we interact with food. In an experiment on healthy and unhealthy foods, using the color red near food helped to reduce the amount of unhealthy food people ate.[55] Interestingly, the color didn't have quite as strong an effect in reducing consumption of healthy food. It's likely that when we hear the word *healthy* we think that we can eat unlimited amounts. That association may be stronger than the associations we have with the color red.

In another study on the color red, consumers took longer to make a decision about a food with a red label than a blue — which suggested that a different cognitive progress was taking place: the mind was slowing down at the sight of the color.[56] And other studies have also shown a strong effect, "red for stop, green for go," when we see those colors in daily life.[57]

Why not make that reaction work to your advantage? Using the color red is an easy way to tap into an automatic response that is already encoded into our brains.

Hangry to Happy

Red plates. In a study that looked at the use of red, blue, and white plates, people ate the least off of red.[58] In other words, the red subconsciously slowed them down. But you don't have to stop there. Think about using red cups, red utensils, and red napkins, too!

Green for go. In a study of candy bars labeled in red or green, people believed the ones labeled in green must be healthier.[59] And it's also been proven that we think "go" or "healthy" when we see the color green.[60] So put healthy snacks in green containers, or use a green snack bowl for healthy snacks on the kitchen counter to help you "go" for these snacks!

Mindful smile. Want to remind yourself to eat a healthy snack? In an inner-city elementary school, green smiley face emoticons were placed on healthy foods in the lunch line. The amount of white milk purchased rose from 7.4 percent baseline to 17.9 percent when the smiley faces were added. And chocolate milk consumption fell by about 20 percent, too. Not only that, but there was a significant increase in vegetable purchases. So draw a smiley face on a Post-it note, and stick it on any mindful snack you would like to make sure you eat.[61] Or take a marker and draw a smile right on the box or wrapper!

HANGER FREE #17: EATING ON THE ROAD

"My husband and I used to fight all the time when we traveled. Our vacations are usually very active, with biking and hiking. If we don't pack enough snacks, a pleasant scenic ride can instantly turn into a bickering match—mostly because he and I are just hangry. I've learned the hard way—packing snacks has saved our vacations!"

When I travel . . .

a) I struggle to find healthy options while traveling.
b) I often can't find what I want to eat and waste a lot of time looking.
c) I choose restaurants ahead of time on the internet.
d) I pack a lot of snacks so I can wait until I find just the right option.

Are you going on a trip anytime soon? If so, one of the things that's probably crossed your mind is food: "What am I going to eat while I'm gone?"

Whether it is a vacation to Disney World or a business trip, traveling causes a lot of eating anxiety for my clients. They worry that they will overeat when they eat out. But they also worry about missing out. If they're going to Boston, they want to be able to eat the clam chowder. If they're going to Italy, they want to eat the pasta.

My clients also struggle with how to eat mindfully on business trips. Research shows that people who travel often for business struggle more with their eating and gain more weight than others.[62]

When we travel, our routine is altered, and our options drastically change. For one thing, our schedules can be all over the place. Our sleep patterns often shift when traveling, which leads to an increase in appetite and often jet lag. Traveling is stressful on your body, which can lead to stress eating. I know I personally never sleep well when I am not in my own bed. And when traveling, our food options are often unfamiliar or limited. It's sometimes a game of *eat this rest stop pizza now because I am starving* or *take my chances that there is a better option down the road ten miles*. It's hard enough to decide what to eat on your own home turf—and even harder when we're away from home.

Day trips can be just as tough as longer ones. My family once went on a road trip to the Columbus Zoo, about an hour and a half away from our home. The excitement of seeing the animals threw off our eating schedule entirely. At one point, I saw my children fade and begin to complain. So I sat them down in the shade and gave them a brief snack. It felt like a hassle to take the time to do that. But as soon as they had some food and a break from the sun, they perked right up. The rest of the time was devoid of whining, which was well worth the investment.

Traveling doesn't have to lead to hanger meltdowns, for our kids, or for us. We plan all kinds of details when we take a trip, from packing to travel logistics. To manage our hunger, we just need to plan for it, too.

Hangry to Happy

Portable, nutrient–dense snacks. Travel often includes a lot of movement and activity. When you need energy for a long hike, a shopping trip, a drive in the mountains or day at the beach, feed your body with filling, protein-rich foods such as nuts, cheese, jerky, protein bars, and almond or peanut butter.

Hit the grocery store. Wherever you go, there's probably a grocery store. So don't just stop at restaurants along the way. Find a grocery store, and hit their salad bar or produce section and load up on snacks.

Play car games. When we're bored on the road, we tend to mindlessly eat. So keep your mind busy in the car by playing games or listening to audiobooks.

Freeze water bottles. Hydration helps you to avoid travel lag and junk-food cravings from boredom in the car. And frozen or cool water bottles can double as massagers: put one behind your neck in the car or on an airplane and roll your shoulders over the bottle or under your feet to cool down. When they defrost, take a sip!

Use an app. Before you leave, plot out your food options with apps such as AroundMe or Yelp, which can help you locate healthier restaurants on the go.

Try protein powder. Traveling requires a lot of energy! Bring some protein powder to add to your yogurt, oatmeal, milk, etc.

Supplement. Traveling can be hard on the body. Even one lost hour of sleep can increase your appetite. Be sure to bring along your vitamins and melatonin to help keep your sleep and appetite in check.

SUMMARY OF HANGER-FREE HOMES AND HANGOUTS

Whether you are cooking dinner at home, munching at the office, or dining in a restaurant, *where* you eat and *what* type of dining utensils and plates you use affect whether you eat mindfully or not. We may wish that we eat just when we are hungry. Period. But that is not the truth, or the reality, of the situation.

After you read this chapter, it's likely that you'll start to take a mindful look around you. Take the time to spin around, 360 degrees, to look at where you are eating and what you are eating on. Remember that these factors can be sneaky. Sometimes they help you to eat mindfully, and other times they don't. The key is to pay attention to them!

Checklist for a Hanger-Free Home and Hangout:

___ I'm mindful of what I eat off of (plates, cups, napkins).

___ I strategically place food and put it away.

___ I place food out of reach to prevent grazing.

___ I am mindful of how I eat while I watch TV.

___ I don't eat in front of a screen.

___ I am aware of when I snack and I am intentional about it.

___ I use helpful cues to eat mindfully and to stop mindless eating.

___ I eat mindfully when I travel.

Hear Your Hunger

When my clients talk about hunger, the visual image that pops into my mind is hunger personified as an annoying neighbor who keeps knocking on their door day after day. Every day, this neighbor keeps coming back, asking for something. But not always the same thing. Some days, they hem and haw at the door, not sure exactly what they want. Other days, they know exactly what they are seeking, such as a hammer to help them with a household project. So you run off and get the hammer for them. But sometimes, after you've brought the hammer back for them, they say, "That's isn't what I really wanted. Do you have a screwdriver?" Kind of like when you eat a peanut butter sandwich and then say, "No, I really wanted mac and cheese."

Typically, people would like to ignore this persistent and pesky neighbor. Often, my clients similarly want to pretend that they don't hear their hunger knocking. Maybe if they ignore hunger, it will go away on its own. But when we ignore hunger, it just knocks louder. Your stomach grumbles. You get more irritable. Avoiding hunger's knock is not the best option.

Sometime hunger's knocking makes people mad. They get fed up. "What the heck do you want now?" they want to yell. They're irritated to have to figure out what hunger wants. And choosing what to eat feels like a pain in the neck.

Other times, people get very invested in trying to make hunger happy instead of just content. We decide we have to have the perfect thing to eat, not just something that is satisfying enough. And while we're trying to think of the perfect thing, we descend into hanger without realizing it.

Instead of ignoring, placating, or fighting off hunger, think about inviting hunger in to chat so you can get to know each other. This way, you won't get frustrated next time. And you can even begin to anticipate what hunger needs and have it waiting at the front door every time you hear a knock.

Hunger isn't bad or good. It's just information from your body. And we need to learn how to understand it. In this section, you learn how to assess your hunger level. Step toward it. Get up close and personal with it. Understand how YOUR hunger happens. And make hanger transform into a happier you.

HEAR YOUR HUNGER #18: HANG UP ON YOUR HANGRY VOICE

"When my husband suggests making broccoli with dinner, my automatic reaction is to narrow my eyes, shake my head, and say, 'Yuck! No way.' I don't even really think about it; I've always just hated broccoli. I'm starting to realize that I'm often not open to the idea of new foods, particularly ones that I have found bland in the past. The Hanger Management program made me more aware of how my internal dialogue—that voice in my head that steers my food choices—is very powerful."

In my internal dialogue about food...

a) I don't talk to myself about my food choices. I just eat.
b) I do a lot of internal debating with myself about what to eat.
c) I consciously think through my food options.
d) I am very mindful about how I think about my food choices.

Language matters. The way we talk to ourselves about the food we eat has a powerful effect on the way we eat.

One of the reasons we have negative feelings about food is because the language of dieting is so negative—even violent. Think about it.

"Slash your hunger!"

"Conquer cravings!

"Squash your appetite."

Language like that hardly makes dieting—or eating at all—seem like a happy activity.

Whether we realize it or not, we're constantly talking to ourselves about what we eat. So I encourage my clients to be mindful of that little inner voice with its ongoing commentary. Because that dialogue has power. If we say to ourselves, "Eww! The asparagus looks gross!" there's no way we're going to try it, no matter how good it might be.

To shift out of our old mindless eating routines, we can make two important but simple shifts in the way we talk to ourselves about food.

First, I teach my clients to rethink how they use the word *full*. My clients often talk about wanting to feel "full." But what do they mean? Is it just a physical feeling—the extension of the stomach or heaviness? Or does it mean something more? Instead of thinking in terms of being "full," I suggest my clients start thinking about what makes them feel content—satisfied, pleased, and accepting of how things are. And I encourage them to notice that contentment has a mental component to it, beyond just the physical. It's important to understand this, because we don't always feel full when we are. It can take our body's sensors several minutes after we eat to feel full. By the time my clients feel the actual physical feelings of fullness in their stomach, they have often overeaten.

To transform their idea of fullness, I ask my clients to imagine an empty paper shopping bag. Then I tell them to mentally imagine filling it until it is full. They often tell me that they imagine filling it completely, with items popping out of the top.

Then I say, "Now imagine filling the bag so that it feels comfortable to carry." The bag they imagine this time looks much different. They leave some room and don't feel pressure to use every nook and cranny. The same can be true of the way we fill our stomachs.

The second important shift in thinking is to start being mindful of how we talk about certain foods, particularly healthy foods.

When my clients talk, I listen closely. I pay attention to every word they use to talk about food. Do they speak about it in happy terms: *enjoy, savor, appreciate, felt great, empowered, fueled up*? Or do they talk about food in negative terms: *boring, bland, hate, drab, uncomfortable, shouldn't, bad*? Sometimes the communication isn't even verbal: often, my clients crinkle their noses when they talk about certain foods, such as vegetables.

My clients' word choices give me a glimpse into their inner voices. And when we recognize what that voice is saying, we can start to use its power in positive ways.

In one study, researchers used different categories of language to label green beans. The basic label was *green beans*. A different label emphasized that the beans were healthy, but reminded diners that they should be restricting their diets: "light 'n' low-carb green beans and shallots." Still another gave more positive, healthful spin on the dish: "healthy energy-boosting green beans and shallots." A final label advertised the dish as an indulgence: "sweet sizzlin' green beans and crispy shallots." Diners chose the vegetables with indulgent labeling 25 percent more than basic labeling, 35 percent more than healthy positive labeling, and 41 percent more than healthy restrictive labeling. Interestingly, diners seemed to prefer the basic label to either of the labels that emphasized the health benefits of the vegetables.[63] Unfortunately, sometimes healthy food gets negatively stereotyped as tasting bad.

The way we talk about our food matters. Be mindful of the way you think, and you'll transform the way you eat.

Hangry to Happy

Mind your language. Listen to the way you talk to yourself about what and how you eat. Don't do anything but listen. I have people imagine their hangry voice on one shoulder and their healthy, happy one on the other. As you make your food choices, take note of which voice is talking. What does your hangry voice sound like—a grouchy old man or a snippy, critical commentator? How about the voice that encourages you to eat healthy, like a supportive friend or a kind parent?

Affirm yourself. The language my clients often use at first communicates loud and clear that they don't believe that they can do it. They say things like, "I have failed so many times at eating mindfully." Or "I can't." Or "I have no self-control." Research shows that such language keeps people stuck in old habits.[64] But studies also show that self-affirming language helps people to have more conscious control over their choices. So start replacing negative thoughts with positive ones, like "It's hard, but I can do this. I am persistent and can do anything when I try."[65]

Redefine *full.* Instead of eating to be full, set your intention to continue eating until you no longer feel hungry. Then ask yourself, "Do I feel content?"

Have fun! A great way to be open to new foods is to have fun with the descriptors you use, as suggested by the study I discussed above. Whenever you eat, choose three fun adjectives to apply to whatever you're eating. For example: "My silky, smooth, decadent Greek yogurt snack." Did you smile when you read this description? Words can make us happy!

HEAR YOUR HUNGER #19: ANTICIPATING HANGER

"I try to anticipate when my family will be hungry each night so I can feed them dinner at just the right time. If I wait too long, they start snacking and rummaging around the kitchen, ruining their appetite. If I serve dinner too soon, no one eats anything and I feel frustrated. I wish we could eat at 6:00 on the dot. However, we are juggling eating with daily events like sports practice or my wife coming home later than expected from work due to traffic."

I usually realize that I'm hungry...

a) when it's too late and I'm in the depths of hunger.
b) when I start to feel twinges of irritation and know it's from being hungry.
c) as soon as I feel hunger. I recognize it immediately.
d) rarely. I anticipate what time I am likely to need to eat.

Restaurants and food companies bank on being able to understand how and when we tend to get hungry. And they use this knowledge of our appetites to their advantage.

For example, McDonald's partnered with Google to use real-time data to drive McDelivery orders during the World Cup. Working with the media agency OMD Hong Kong, McDonald's harnessed Google's real-time trigger program for advertisers and a data-management platform to anticipate times during matches when fans would become hungry and to push ads enticing them to place orders.[66, 67]

The "hungry moments" were calculated based on the insight that football fans get hungry when they're excited. So ads were pushed at the beginning of the game, halftime, the end of the game, and whenever a goal was scored.

Advertisers know that anticipating our hunger is key to getting us to buy food. But I've found in my practice that anticipating our own hunger can do the opposite: help us to make better choices about what and when we eat. Mindfully anticipating hunger is one of our best defenses against hanger.

Most of us learn how to anticipate problems in our lives. We can't tell always tell the future, but we can predict things that are likely to go wrong, based on our experience. For example, I give presentations on mindful eating all around the world. There are two big challenges that come up over and over again. The technology doesn't work or the host doesn't have enough handouts. And when either of these things happen, the presentation comes to a screeching halt. So I've learned to anticipate these problems and bring solutions—a backup copy of my presentation and extra handouts.

It's harder for most of us to anticipate our hunger. Sometimes, we're great at anticipating the hunger of people who are close to us, especially our partners and kids. We see the signs a mile away—a spouse wandering around the kitchen, a child starting to snack on anything handy, or the first inklings of irritation.

Seeing our own hunger coming can be much more challenging. My clients have great plans for dealing with their hunger, but then a snag in the day will send them spiraling in a different direction. They're running late, so they don't stop to pick up that snack they planned to keep on hand. Things are busy at work, so they can't leave the building to pick up food the way they usually do.

It's not just a matter of anticipating your hunger, but of making a plan. I see that even in my own life. I've spent years paying attention to my own hunger. I know about how long it generally takes me to get hungry. And I know my hanger vulnerability moments, like Thursday mornings when I'm up earlier than usual, move more, and see many more people in counseling. Since I know it's coming every week, I try to plan ahead. But if I don't think about what might go wrong with my plan, I'm still likely to get hangry if there's a snag in my day.

To prevent that takes an extra step: thinking about what hiccups might happen and taking steps to make sure you stay on track, even when the day is full of surprises.

Hangry to Happy

Interview your hunger. To lay a solid plan against hanger, take the time to think about what you know about when you are most likely to get hangry—and what you can do about it. Ask yourself a series of *W* questions.

> *Where* do I tend to get hungry the most? At work? At home? On the road? Someplace else?

When do I tend to get hungry? Mornings? Evenings? Weekends? Certain days?

Why do I tend to get hungry when I do? Am I bored? Busy?
Going too long between snacks or meals?

What are my hungry signals? Do I start to think about food?
Do I get irritable? Do I get lethargic?

Use the hanger-alert system. Preventing hunger means
staying one step ahead of it. And the good news is that our body
does give us some warning signs. Before we get hungry, we feel
twinges. But many of us wait until hunger hits us over the head,
and we're starving. By then, it's painfully clear that we're in need
of food, and fast.

As you move through your day, take time to stop every hour
or so and notice how hungry you feel. Take notes on how you
feel from hour to hour—or whenever you're able to take a
moment to be mindful of your hunger through the day—and
use the rating system below.

Hanger Alert System

1) Content: No Need to Eat
Experiencing your normal resting state
Not perceiving hunger at the moment
Not thinking about food

2) Early Hunger: Becoming Mindful of Hunger
Considering food options
Beginning to notice signs of hunger

3) Hungry: Eat NOW
Thinking a lot about food
Planning what to eat
Needing a snack or meal

Feeling lower energy

4) Famished: Urgent!

Feeling very low energy

Growing irritable

Experiencing stomach growling

Craving food

Seeking food

5) Too Late! Hanger Alert!

Having trouble focusing or concentrating

Feeling less patience

Overreacting to small things

Finding thinking and memory cloudy

Developing headaches

Experiencing lethargy

Letting minor stressors create irritation

Feeling that everything is a big deal and feels hard

Snapping at people or saying things that aren't like you

Regretting decisions later

Make a hanger plan. Ask yourself, "What is my plan for each level of the alert system?" Write down what you can do at each stage. For example, "If I am at the Urgent level, I will stop what I am doing immediately and have a substantial snack of X."

Troubleshoot your plan. Ask yourself what could go wrong with your plan. List three things that could cause a snag in your day: A sick kid? A meeting that runs over? A business prospect who won't stop chatting about his next big project? What can you do to get by? The answer to this is often not an ideal option, but something that will work in a pinch—something that will tide you over for the moment if all else goes wrong.

HEAR YOUR HUNGER #20: COPING WITH HANGXIETY

"Oh my gosh, I am STARVING! My husband says that when I feel hungry, I always feel the urge to announce it to the world. He has a point. I do say it like it's an emergency. It's almost like I panic a little. Now what do I do?"

When I get hungry I . . .

a) think "Oh, no! I'm hungry. Now what? I have no idea what to eat."
b) feel anxious and begin to fret about what to eat.
c) think about what sounds really good and yummy. I day-dream about this for a while.
d) calmly come up with a plan based on what food is available and sounds good to me.

I remember going to an afternoon wedding outdoors in late June. Like many weddings, there was a big gap between the ceremony and the following reception. I knew my husband would be sweating in his navy suit, adding to his discomfort level. And I started to get something I call "hangxiety" about what we would do between the wedding and the reception. It was too long not to eat anything. And what if we got to the reception and we didn't get anything to eat for two more hours, until it was an appropriate dinner time? Also, it was likely that the drinks from cocktail hour would make me sleepy without something solid in my stomach. I wanted to enjoy the wedding. But I knew that he would be a grumpy mess if I didn't figure out a solid strategy.

Many of my clients struggle with hangxiety, too.

Simply put, hangxiety is when hunger makes you feel anxious. Sometimes you might be just a little anxious. You might feel a little flutter in your heart or fret a little bit about what there is to eat: "What do I have? There is nothing good." Other times, hangxiety can lead to a full-on meltdown. And it may not happen only when you're hungry. For some of my clients, even thinking about the fact that they might get hungry can give them hangxiety.

Hangxiety can be so intense that people just don't want to deal with it. And research indicates that this makes sense from a biological perspective. In caveman times, hunger was a huge, real problem. It meant you had to go hunting or scavenging. And if you didn't find something, you might go hungry for days. In a modern context, around the world and in places close to all our homes, people still go hungry because food is not available. Images of children in war-torn countries or in natural disasters haunt us. So in some contexts, hunger is associated with very real emergencies, crises, or famines. Don't be hard on yourself if getting hungry makes you feel panicky. That feeling is rooted in something real.

What brings on hangxiety? Some hangxiety comes from the fact that once you realize you're hungry, you have to make a decision. And knowing what to do isn't always easy.

The bad news is that people who feel hangxiety often eat as a way to manage their anxiety level. They nibble and munch to calm their nerves. And that's not always the best decision— though it is understandable.

What I have learned from working with people who have anxiety—any kind of anxiety—is that having an escape plan reduces your anxiety tremendously. For example, someone who is anxious about going to a graduation party can get a lot of relief by plotting out how they can gracefully leave if they feel overwhelmed. And because they know they can leave, they often don't. Just knowing they have a plan helps them relax and enjoy the whole situation more.

The same can apply with hangxiety. If you have a strategy in place for avoiding hangxiety, you can skip both anxious eating and being paralyzed by what to do when hunger hits!

Hangry to Happy

Give yourself a break. If you get hangxiety when you're hungry, that's okay. Remind yourself that the feeling of hunger is a normal and natural feeling. Don't waste time feeling bad when you could be thinking about what to do next.

Get comfortable with hunger. Work on getting comfortable with little bits of hunger. A twinge of hunger might make you uncomfortable, but it won't really hurt you. Sit with it, so you can learn from it. Notice where the discomfort of hunger arises in your body. Experiment with different time frames between eating to see what various levels of hunger feel like.

Learn the difference. Sometimes we confuse hunger and anxiety. So pay attention to when and where you feel anxiety in your body. What lets you know you're feeling anxious? Do you breathe fast? Clench your teeth? Something else? Pay attention, and make sure you know the difference between anxiety and hunger. Anxiety shows up in more ways—such as a rapid heartbeat and shallow breathing. Hunger is mostly centered in your stomach, energy level, mood, and thoughts about food.

Have a hangxiety plan. Create a decision tree about what you can do to manage hunger when you feel it, or what I call the "If X, then Y" plan. Make a list of possible scenarios and how to manage them. For example, one of my personal plans is, *If I get hungry for a snack while driving, I will pull over and eat the bag of almonds*

I keep stashed in my armrest. I don't worry about getting hungry, because I know a handful of these almonds is a healthy option to get me by for the moment. Along with your plans to deal with hunger, make a plan for when you feel anxious. Start by taking slow, deep breaths to calm down your fight-or-flight response — then decide what will work best to calm your anxiety.

HEAR YOUR HUNGER #21: BE THE HUNGER WHISPERER

"My schedule is crazy hectic. I am constantly running at a breakneck pace to get things done."

When it comes to paying attention to my hunger...

a) I am so busy that I don't really pay attention to my hunger.
b) I often know when I am hungry — and ignore it.
c) I try to check in with my body to know if I am really hungry or if I am full.
d) I know exactly when I am hungry and when I am getting full.

The art of mindful eating comes down to this: listening.

Listen to your hunger. Sometimes we hear our hunger loud and clear. We take it seriously. We empathize with how we feel and try to make it better. We realize it's been a long day, and that we're craving something warm and hearty.

However, sometimes we don't listen at all. We ignore very loud and clear signs of hunger because we are busy, or we just don't want to hear it. Instead of responding to our hunger, our inner voice says, "Oh, just hush up!"

Listening to your hunger is no different than listening to your significant other. The other day my client told me a story about her husband. In the morning, she had told him the time and place to pick up the kids. He appeared to be listening. He even nodded and said, "Have a great day." But around three o'clock, he called her in a bit of panic. "What did you say about the kids? When and where do I have to pick them up?" She'd had only half of his attention earlier.

My clients are often the same when hunger starts talking to them. While they are bulldozing along in life, the lines of communication with their bodies are not always open—or they're only half-listening. Then, when it's time to act, they are clueless about what to do. When we don't respond to hunger, the body hits mute—for a while. But then the hunger comes back, even stronger. One of my client's favorite mantras is, "If you listen to your body whisper, you don't have to hear it scream."

Your body is giving you messages all the time. For example, if you bump your arm, your body sends you pain cues. You respond with an action, often something like rubbing the sore spot. But it's not just any action. When we're in pain, we usually try a compassionate and soothing action. We are often way more responsive to other physical sensations than we are to our hunger.

Some of my clients who now listen really intently to their bodies learned the hard way. They are the ones who have pushed their bodies to the point of injury. Now they realize they pushed right past their bodies telling them to stop, and they paid the price. Often, people who have food allergies have learned to listen to their bodies as well. I have a friend, Lila, who has a dairy allergy. If she has any bit of dairy, she vomits instantly because her body thinks it is a foreign invader. She has to be very mindful of what she eats or she will end up feeling awful!

To ward off hanger, we need to learn to turn the volume of our hunger back on. When my clients learn to mindfully listen to their hunger, something happens: they respond with thoughtful, mindful action.

Hangry to Happy

The trick to hearing your hunger is to begin to listen with a mindful, empathetic ear—not just to hear that you are hungry, but to respond with an understanding of what you need, right now. Take a look at these levels of listening:

Mindful Listening. Listening with both the heart and mind. *"I'm hungry. I know. That's uncomfortable. I feel low energy. What do I need right now? Something to perk up my energy level."*

Focused Listening. Paying attention mentally to what your body is telling you about your hunger but ignoring any associated emotions. *"I'm just hungry."*

Selective Listening. Hearing only the parts of the conversation that interest you. *"I could use some food. I only want candy!"*

Pretend Listening. Giving the impression you are listening, but not really taking the situation seriously. *"Yeah, yeah, I know I'm hungry. I'll get to it later."*

Ignoring. Making no effort to listen. You act as if your hunger doesn't matter and other things are more important. *"I shouldn't be hungry. I just ate three hours ago."* Ask yourself, "On what level am I listening to my hunger right now?" Then use these tips to start mindful, empathetic listening to your hunger.

Slow down. *"The quieter you become, the more you can hear."* —*Ram Dass*

When your car engine is revving, you can't hear much of

anything else. To quiet your own engine, slow down and spend a moment taking inventory of how you feel. Pick at least three times a day to pause and eavesdrop on your body.

Learn your cues. Think about your hunger as the check-engine light in your car. Your body communicates with you all the time. For instance, when you are tired, your body sends you some clear signs. Your eyes begin to get heavy and your breathing starts to slow down. As your fatigue escalates, you yawn. What are your signs that you're hungry? How do they change as your hunger increases?

Try a yoga pose. If you're having trouble hearing your body, yoga is a great way to get to know your physical self. Try this yoga pose that you can do sitting in a chair. Begin seated with your knees bent 90 degrees and your feet flat. Press down from your heels, trying not to move your feet in toward your chair or use your arms, and make your way up to a standing position. Once you're standing, slowly sit straight back down, refraining from leaning forward and/or shifting your hips to one side or the other. Repeat five to ten times. Bring awareness to your feet against the floor, your balance, and the tension in the back of your thighs as you slowly sit down. This pose is helpful to center and ground you at a table before you eat. You can do this yoga pose or *any* pose that speaks to you. The point is that yoga helps us to be present in our bodies.

HEAR YOUR HUNGER #22: OVERCOMING HANGER OBSTACLES

"I'm busy. This is what I tell myself about why I don't eat healthier. It's true — between managing school, work, and trying to see my boyfriend. But sometimes, when I am radically honest with myself, I know that I

make time for everything else in my life. But eating healthier just slips right down to the bottom of my priority list."

When I try to follow through on my plans to eat healthier...

a) it's almost impossible. It never seems to happen, even if I want it to.
b) it takes a lot of effort for me. I wish I followed through more frequently.
c) some days it happens, and other days it doesn't.
d) I have got the hang of it, and I eat mindfully most of the time.

"But..."

It's a tiny word—and an extremely powerful word.

But...I'm too busy to eat.

But...I'm too stressed.

But...it's such a hassle.

What I have learned as a psychologist is that people *want* to eat healthy. We earnestly wish to take care of ourselves.

There are just so many "buts" that stand in the way.

I haven't met a person yet who says they aren't interested in improving their diet. No one likes the feeling of being overly hungry or turning into a hangry, not-so-pleasant version of themselves. Or getting stuck in cycles of hunger, undereating, and overeating.

Many of us struggle because some kind of real barrier stands in our way.

Where I live, for example, many of my clients drive more than twenty miles to get to the nearest store. So even having healthy food on hand requires time, planning, and money. Other barriers are emotional, like stress or fear of change. Being tired or overwhelmed can make swinging by a fast-food place much more tempting than going to the grocery store. These are the emotional obstacles I see most frequently at my office. They're less visible than the physical barriers but just as real.

According to a study that spanned fifteen European nations, the biggest barriers people reported to healthy eating were lack of time, irregular work schedules, and a preference for certain foods over others.[68] Do these ring a bell for you?

I see those factors at play in my own practice. And perhaps because I'm a psychologist, I also see something else: how much our emotions can affect healthy eating.

For many of my clients, the emotional obstacles boil down to these issues: busy, blue, and bothersome.

Busy: They feel too busy to cook, shop, or prep food. Other things in life just take a higher priority.

Blue: They feel stressed out. They do a lot of emotional eating. When they feel stressed or overwhelmed, it's hard to allocate energy toward eating healthy.

Bothersome: Healthy eating feels like a hassle. Changing their status quo habits takes a lot of work, which isn't always easy.

The first thing I have my clients do is identify which obstacle to healthy eating stands in the way most often. Then I have them drill down deep, to get to the nitty-gritty details—which is where the solutions can be found.

For example, one of my clients identified her primary barrier as busyness. She focused on everything around her and took care of everyone else. Managing her own hunger was the last thing on her mind. Hearing herself say "But I have to take care of... first" caused her plans to eat mindfully to come to a screeching halt.

Once my client knew her "buts," she was able to start work-ing on turning hanger into happiness. She said it was almost like having traffic updates on her phone, giving her information on delays, accidents, and road closures. One second of checking in on traffic let her know what was ahead and helped her plot a good course, without getting caught up in the frustration of delays that stopped her in her tracks.

Instead of wasting energy stewing about her busyness and hanger, she started to focus her energy on how to fit healthy eat-ing into her life in convenient ways, like ordering snack foods online to avoid the store, having the grocery store deliver grocer-ies to her door, and using a slow cooker.

Hangry to Happy

Turn *but* into *and*. To turn from hangry to happy, you have to get past the "but..." voice in your head. Acknowledge the *but*s. Don't try to talk yourself out of thinking them. Instead, just acknowledge the voice and empathize with whatever it is that's tripping you up. Understanding your barrier can help you to brainstorm about what to do about it. Reframe the *but* into an *and: "I want to eat more mindfully AND I am really busy."*

Do what you are already doing—more mindfully. Instead of feeling that you have to adopt a new routine, just com-mit to doing what you are *already doing,* but in a more mindful way. For example, if you are eating a snack, do it mindfully by turning off your phone while you eat. If you are going to have a piece of chocolate, do it more mindfully by eating it slowly. These things *don't take even a second more of time,* but they shift the way you eat. If you are feeling that eating mindfully is just too big of a bother, this tip is perfect for you.

HEAR YOUR HUNGER #23: PHANTOM FULLNESS

"I eat a bagel for breakfast, which I feel is huge and should keep me completely full all day long. But frustratingly, I get hungry again right away. I think 'What is wrong with me?'"

When I eat...

a) I feel hungry again almost immediately.
b) I seem to get hungry again quickly.
c) I feel satisfied for a while.
d) I am satisfied until it's time for my next snack or meal.

My client Julie was describing what it was like for her to eat an oversized blueberry muffin. "This should really keep me full for a long time," she told herself as she ate.

But poof!

An hour later, she was ravenous again.

Many of my clients experience this. I call it "phantom fullness."

They eat something, even something that seems substantial, but their feeling of fullness quickly vanishes into thin air. What they're eating does very little to satisfy them and keep their hunger at bay. So hanger pops up all the time.

At first, my clients like Julie blame themselves and their bodies. They say, "I shouldn't be hungry again. What is wrong with me? How could I get hungry again this quickly?"

When my clients and I talk about what they've been eating, often we uncover something interesting. They are frequently eating foods that are infamous for creating phantom fullness.

Research indicates that some foods are processed by the body much more quickly than other foods. And foods like that are a direct path to hanger.

In one study, women were given one of three different afternoon snacks. All three of them contained 160 calories. The three options were high-protein yogurt, high-fat crackers, and high-fat chocolate.[69]

You might think that because they all contain the same calories, they'd all affect the body about equally. But that's not what researchers found. The women who ate the yogurt were less hungry during the afternoon than those who ate the chocolate. And women who ate the yogurt got hungry later than the other women: 20 minutes later than the women who ate crackers, and a whole 30 minutes later than the women who ate chocolate.

The choice of snacks even affected what the women chose to eat for dinner later. The women who ate yogurt consumed less at dinner than the women who'd had crackers or chocolate.

What a person eats affects how they feel both in the moment and later on, down the line. And when my clients begin to really tune in to this factor and get to know which snacks keep phantom fullness away, they begin to eat foods that make them feel happy, not hungry.

Hangry to Happy

My clients get to know their bodies well, to a T. They learn which foods affect their mood and how full they feel. And when this connection is crystal clear, it starts to change how they choose food.

To get to know what keeps *you* from getting phantom fullness, try an experiment on yourself similar to the study described above.

The 3 Experiment: Choose three different snacks: For example, you might try a high-protein one (such as cheese, nuts, lunch meat, or yogurt), a healthy snack (piece of fruit or raw veggies), and a treat snack (chocolate, potato chips, candy). Or just pick three of your most common favorite snacks. Eat each of them on different days.

Take notes. What do you notice about how these different snacks affect your happiness or hangriness level *3* minutes later, *30* minutes later, and *3* hours later?

HEAR YOUR HUNGER #24: COPING WITH "I WANT THAT!"

"I walk past a macaron shop every day on my way to work. I see rows and rows of these multicolored cookies. For the next block, I think about them, wishing I'd had time to stop. I'd keep thinking about them all day long. Then I'd make sure I walked past the shop on the way home so I could stop and buy some."

When it comes to the way food looks to me . . .

a) I see something tasty to eat and I immediately want it.
b) I often eat foods just because they look good.
c) I think about how something will taste and how much it will fill me up.
d) I know what foods taste good to me and fill me up, and I eat them mindfully.

I have a client who loves chocolate.
She loves it so much that she thought she had to stop eating it.

So my advice surprised her. "Start taking your appetite for chocolate seriously," I told her. "Go ahead and have a piece a day."

So she started to eat a piece a day, on "doctor's orders." She started looking forward to the daily treat.

And she got another surprise. Eating her daily chocolate made it easier for her to pass up other treats that she didn't really love. Because she knew she was going to have a taste of chocolate every day, she no longer felt the need to eat everything that looked appetizing.

We use the words *appetite* and *hunger* as if they're the same thing.

But they're not.

And one of the important tips I teach my clients is to tell the difference between them.

Hunger is biological in nature. It involves *internal* cues such as a rumbling stomach. And it's triggered by measurable chemical factors, like blood sugar and hormones.

Appetite, on the other hand, is the desire to eat as a result of external cues. When we see, smell, or think about food, we may develop an appetite. You've probably experienced this yourself: when you smell warm bread in the oven or see a commercial for a food you love, suddenly you feel like eating something, even after you have eaten a meal and are satisfied.

Appetite can also be triggered by routine. My clients talk about suddenly wanting a certain food because they are in a particular place or situation. For example, when the country fair rolls around again each year in September in my town, many of my clients begin to express a desire for elephant ears. They express no appetite for the fried and sugary confections during the rest of the year. It's the circumstance—having the fair come to town—that drives the desire.

Our appetite isn't the same as hunger, but it's still powerful. My clients often talk about the ways in which their appetite sometimes overcomes their hunger drive. Once their appetite is engaged, it's all about what they want, not how hungry they are. They often feel as if they are at the mercy of their appetite, which leads them this way and that. My client Clare talks a lot about orange cookies. As soon as she thinks about them, she says, "I can't get them out of my mind."

Some of my clients try to fight their hunger and their appetite. If you do this, you aren't alone. But telling yourself to ignore your appetite is like telling yourself to stop breathing. Or telling yourself "I'll only breathe three times a day."

The problem is that when we feed our appetite instead of our hunger, we often end up feeling hangry. But the same thing is true if we try to ignore our appetite completely. If we "just say no" to the things that stimulate our appetite, it's like trying to ignore a crying baby. Our appetite does need attention. But it needs the right kind of attention. You can get a baby to stop crying when you meet his or her need in just the right way. The good news is that the same is true with your appetite.

Hangry to Happy

My motto with clients is: *"Mindfully feed your appetite."* When you give yourself permission to feed your appetite in mindful ways, you no longer feel the need to respond to it every time it says "I want!"

But learning your appetite takes time — and mindfulness.

Breathe deep. Before you take a bite, take at least six deep breaths. A study showed that taking slow, deep breaths can slow down your heart rate. Female students performed paced breathing while looking at their favorite food on a computer screen. Slow paced breathing appeared to alter the experience of hunger. Relaxing the body = reducing cravings. Wow! Just slowing down your breathing can help you eat more mindfully.[70]

Be honest. Ask yourself if this is your appetite or hunger talking. Is this a *want* or a *need*? Both are fine, just be clear on which one you are dealing with.

Get conscious of your appetite triggers. What triggers your appetite? Is it the sight of food? Commercials? Smells? Circumstances? Does the heavenly scent of baked goods prompt cravings, or are you someone who eats with their eyes? Food that looks amazing makes you want it! Some triggers you can avoid. Others you can't. But just knowing your sensory triggers can help you anticipate which ones will likely set you off, so you can be ready for them!

Eat mindfully. When you eat the foods that stimulate your appetite, eat mindfully. Do whatever you need to enjoy every bite. Sit down. Stop whatever else you are doing. And eat slowly, to get the most pleasure possible.

Mind the happy benefits. Hedy Kober, an associate professor of psychiatry and psychology at Yale, published a study in the *Proceedings of the National Academy of Sciences* in which her team conducted several experiments to measure the effects of simple cognitive training techniques on eating habits.[71] In one experiment, people read literature on healthy foods and received 15 minutes of training on how to deal with cravings by thinking of how good they would feel if they chose a nutritious, healthy food. Interestingly, focusing on the benefits of what you gain from eating well right now can help you to choose more mindfully.

You can do the same: change the way you eat by thinking about the benefits of eating mindfully. Before you decide what to eat, take a moment to review three benefits to choosing to eat mindfully right *now.*

One immediate benefit for your *mind,* like the fact that you'll feel less distracted or more in control of your choices.

One benefit for your *mood,* like not experiencing regret or feeling more in charge.

One *physical* benefit of eating mindfully, like not feeling bloated or too full.

SUMMARY OF HEAR YOUR HUNGER

Have you ever played the game of telephone? You sit in a circle. One person whispers a story to the next person. That person whispers it to the next person, and so on down the line. The last person recounts the entire story out loud. The final story often has only a funny, vague resemblance to the original story. Along the way, the message gets lost, loosely interpreted, skewed, made up, or simply not heard.

This is similar to what happens to the story we tell ourselves about our hunger. Along the way, the message you hear about your hunger and what you want or need becomes a little fuzzy. On top of that, hearing and listening are two entirely different actions, whether you are listening to your significant other or tuning in to body cues.

Some days you may feel you need earplugs because your hunger is screaming so loudly at you. Other days, you may feel you need a hunger hearing aid to pick up the vague whispers from your body, telling you about your hunger.

The tools in this chapter, including the checklist on the next page, can help you become an expert listener so you can hear what you need to turn your hunger into happiness.

___ I am mindful of the language and words I use to describe the way I eat.

___ I know what emotional barriers stand in the way of eating mindfully.

___ I don't get anxious about feeling hungry or the possibility of hunger.

___ I listen to what my body wants and needs.

___ I stay ahead of my hunger, anticipating when I will be hungry.

___ I pay attention to which foods fill me up and which ones don't.

___ I know the difference between wanting food because it looks good and being genuinely hungry.

___ I am able to respond mindfully rather than react unconsciously to cravings.

Hunger Hypnotizers

This section was challenging for me to write.

Why?

Because I've said over and over again in my books and articles that I don't tell people *what* to eat—and I still don't.

My overall philosophy isn't about this food or that. It's about mindful eating. In my practice, I don't tell people what foods to eat or take off their menu. So I don't want to give the perception that I'm advising something like "You must eat more mushrooms to get vitamin D."

But over the years, my definition of mindful eating has evolved and broadened. It's not just about being aware of your food habits so that you don't mindlessly gobble a sleeve of crackers while watching TV. It's also about being mindful of how certain foods affect your body, mood—and hanger level. When you really tune in to how your body responds to particular foods, you have a much greater ability to harness your hanger.

My client Nicole, for example, is very mindful of how much cheese she eats. She loves every kind of cheese—blue, cheddar, provolone—you name it, she adores it. Although she does not have any dairy or lactose allergy, too much of it doesn't sit well in her stomach. She has told me on many occasions that she pays very close attention to how much cheese is sprinkled on pizza, how many slices of cheese are in a sandwich, and the number of cubes she snacks on. She explained that she completely enjoys a little bit of cheese. But perhaps it's the amount of sodium or saturated fat that can make her to feel sluggish and constipated when she eats a lot of it. Yuck! No one wants to feel that way from food! Thankfully, Nicole is a whiz at knowing how she reacts to certain foods. She uses this knowledge to make sure pleasurable foods don't cause pain.

In this section, your job is twofold. First, you'll learn to understand how foods and nutrients may be supporting or sabotaging your mood and hanger level. Your next job is to experiment. This includes being very tuned in to what happens after you eat food—whether it's a specific food mentioned in this section or something else. Be mindful of how your hunger changes in intensity after you eat. How long does a particular food keep your hunger at bay? How satisfied do you feel after eating it? And most important, does this food make you happy?

About six years ago, my doctor told me that my iron level was low. This wasn't a complete shock to me. I'd been anemic at other points in my life. What did surprise me was that I thought I had stayed on top of it.

I already ate a lot of iron-rich foods. But when I started to boost my iron intake with more of these foods, like leafy greens and meats, something amazing happened. It was like flipping a light switch. My energy level started to rise almost overnight. I had not even realized how much I had been dragging. When my iron levels were low, everything seemed to take more time. But I had chalked it up to more clients on my schedule and having small kids. "Who wouldn't be tired?" I told myself.

When our energy drags, our go-to is often coffee or sugary foods to perk us up. But if your iron level is off, neither one will help at all. And the same is true for any other nutrients you need.

So from here on out, your job is to pay close attention to how your body, hunger, and mood respond to certain foods.

Which foods make you hangry?

And which ones make you happy?

HUNGER HYPNOTIZER #25: HOW TO HANGER-PROOF YOUR DAY

"I am a reformed stress eater. I no longer eat everything I can get my hands on when I've had a crummy day. This is an amazing feat. When I am stressed out, which happens quite a bit, I try to be even more thoughtful about what I eat. The kind of stress I have isn't good for me and tears my body up. I know this because when I have a really terrible day or a huge presentation coming up, I get sick about two days later. My body just gives out from the stress. So I eat lots of oranges, berries, and nuts to help prevent this crash. It's like putting sandbags up to brace against a stress storm."

When I get stressed...

a) I crave comfort food like mac and cheese, tater tots, or chocolate.
b) I care less about my food choices.
c) I completely lose my appetite.

d) I eat food that helps nourish me and prevent the wear and tear of stress.

Every day, I help my clients to stop stress eating.

We work on breaking the complicated "I-feel-stressed-I-want-to-eat-comfort-foods-right-now-to-feel-better" cycle. So often, we use food to soothe uncomfortable and unpleasant feelings, and don't even realize it until after the fact. But then it's too darn late! Other times, we are painfully aware that we are stress eating, and we struggle desperately and unsuccessfully to break the habit.

To break the cycle, I teach my clients and readers to identify when they are truly physically hungry. If they aren't physically hungry, there are natural and healthy alternatives to eating that can also help you to calm down and relax. (See my book *50 Ways to Soothe Yourself Without Food* and the sequel, *50 More Ways to Soothe Yourself Without Food!*)

I always offer a very important caveat, as well. I remind people to *keep eating* when they're stressed. The key is to make sure you're getting foods that fortify your body. Comfort foods make you feel better for a few moments. And honestly, sometimes we just want grilled cheese and french fries—and that's okay. But stress-busting foods can keep your mood from getting worse, and even improve it!

Basically, stress can be like a wrecking ball to your body. It causes inflammation and changes your hormones, which makes you more irritable. So let's try flipping that effect on its head. Eating certain foods that help boost your immune system can help prevent or even repair the stress damage. It's amazing. Food can help build your tolerance to irritation and fortify it to minimize the wear and tear that comes from stress.

When my client Lori, who's a hospice worker, has a stressful week, she makes sure she includes two foods in her diet. She commits to eating more fish that has omega-3. Her choice is backed up by a study from Ohio State University that looked at the impact of an omega-3 diet on stress levels on a group of graduate students before and after exams—a very high-stress time in their lives. Researchers found that students with diets rich in omega-3 fatty acids had 20 percent less anxiety compared to participants who didn't eat omega-rich fish.[72] The food students ate actually reduced their stress.

The second type of food Lori eats during a stressful week is berries, particularly blueberries. She does this because when she is overly stressed, her eyebrows naturally furrow, and she noticed that the furrows were making deep wrinkles in her face.

We talked about a recent study that found a significant relationship between deep forehead wrinkles, stress, and higher risk of dying of a cardiovascular issue. The study found that these deep forehead wrinkles can be a quick and easy screening tool that health-care providers can use if they suspect a patient may be at risk for heart issues. They hypothesize that these wrinkles come from several factors, including stress, high cholesterol, and hypertension.[73] Blueberries are high in antioxidants, which can help prevent oxidative stress, a process in the body that causes cell damage—and wrinkles! So when Lori eats her blueberries, she's helping to rebuild the cell damage caused by stress.

One of my personal favorite foods for stress management is mandarin oranges. Inhaling the scent of an orange for ninety seconds has been shown to cause a significant reaction in the right prefrontal cortex of the brain—which increases comfortable and relaxed feelings.[74] The sweet orange scent decreases the symptoms of anxiety and improves mood. Not to mention that oranges are high in vitamin C, which can help boost your immune system—help we all need when we are stressed out!

During my day, I take a "mindful time-out" and close my door. I sit in my office chair with my orange and peel each segment mindfully. One at a time. Breathing in the sweet citrus smell. I also love cut kiwi and mango, which offer the same benefits, since they also contain vitamin C.

Many people don't utilize the power of food to cope with stress because they believe that they shouldn't eat when stressed. But when we're feeling stressed out and overwhelmed, eating can actually be the best thing for us.

Hangry to Happy

Stress check: Be honest with yourself. Where is your stress level right now? Is it sky-high, through the roof? Do you say to yourself or others daily, "I am so stressed out!" Or maybe you just have some minor annoyances in your life that you can manage. Everyone has some stress. That's to be expected. But if you answered, "It's really high," minding what you eat can help prevent hanger—and reduce the symptoms of stress.

Stress-busting foods. On a stressful day, be sure to arm yourself with stress-busting foods. A mindful snack will help to inoculate the body from cravings and stress eating. And a number of foods help minimize inflammation caused by stress and help you gear up to endure stress that could turn into hanger. Here are a few examples:

Antioxidant-rich Foods: The good news is that these foods are yummy! They include blueberries (which have the highest amount of antioxidants of any berries), cranberries, strawberries, raspberries, spinach, kale, oranges, beans, pecans, and cilantro.

Vitamin E–rich Foods: Sunflower seeds, almonds, hazelnuts, mangoes, avocados, butternut squash, spinach, kiwis, broccoli, and tomatoes are all packed with vitamin E. Vitamin E helps because it has great anti-inflammatory properties, assists immune functioning, and protects your cells from free radicals that break down the body.

Omega-3–rich Foods: Atlantic mackerel, salmon, walnuts, chia seeds, herring, flaxseed, tuna, and egg yolks each contain a big dose of omega-3, which helps reduce the inflammation caused by stress. And avocados are an amazing source of omega-3 as well. To get the benefits, try smashed avocado on whole wheat toast, a simple, filling stress-buster that even young children can make and enjoy.

Pumpkin Seeds: Chock-full of zinc, magnesium, and omega-6, pumpkin seeds are one of my favorite mineral-rich, go-to foods. And if you need a savory fix, reach for pumpkin seeds sprinkled with sea salt or spices.

Teas: Cinnamon tea is clinically shown to regulate blood sugar, making it easier to keep away the hanger. Chamomile tea has been shown to help reduce anxiety and encourage restful sleep. Green tea calms the body during stress. Black tea boasts benefits, too: a study of 75 men found that six weeks of drinking black tea decreased cortisol levels in response to a stressful task, compared to other caffeinated drinks.[75]

Dark Chocolate: More than one study proves that consuming dark chocolate helps reduce cortisol when your body is under stress.[76] Yes, I'm saying an ounce of dark chocolate a day helps keep the stress away!

Bone Broth: Filled with amino acids, bone broth is great for replenishing the body. It increases collagen stores to replace those depleted under stress. And bone broth and good old chicken–noodle soup have anti–inflammatory properties.[77]

HUNGER HYPNOTIZER #26: FOODS THAT KEEP HANGER AT BAY

"I'm in a huge rush in the morning, after I hit snooze repeatedly before class. I tend to skip breakfast all the time, even though I love it. Then it's like a surprise when I am starving by 10:00 a.m., desperate for something to eat."

Do you always start your day with breakfast?

a) I'm just not hungry when I wake up.
b) Nope, coffee will do.
c) I typically forget or don't have time.
d) Yes! Are you kidding? I need it! I just can't function without breakfast.

You know you're "supposed" to eat breakfast. You're well aware of the saying "breakfast is the most important meal of the day." You don't dispute that.

But, gosh darn it, none of that helps when you just rolled out of bed and only have ten minutes to get to a meeting. Or if you aren't really hungry because you mindlessly ate while you were binge-watching TV until 3:00 a.m. Or maybe you just aren't a "breakfast person."

But the old saying is onto something. The drawbacks of skipping breakfast are often serious for your mood. Without breakfast, your blood sugar drops, putting you at risk for low energy and hanger.

In some cases, the consequences of skipping breakfast are even more extreme. My clients who have diabetes have learned firsthand that they can't skip breakfast. They get significantly low blood sugar, called hypoglycemia, which makes them anxious, tired, and shaky.

On the other hand, eating breakfast offers all kinds of benefits. The instant you eat breakfast, good things begin to happen. Research published in the *Journal of Frontiers of Human Neuroscience* shows that eating breakfast helps restore glycogen and stabilizes levels of insulin.[78] And the positive effects of breakfast persist all day. One study shows that women who ate breakfast ate less throughout the day than those who skipped it.[79] In other words, they didn't overeat later because they were well fed from the start.

The most compelling reason for eating breakfast is that it helps you enjoy life more. One study of contemporary dancers looked at what happened when some dancers in the study were given an energy bar to eat, while others fasted with water before ballet class.[80] The study found that dancers who consumed the energy bar had greater peaks in blood-glucose levels than those who fasted. This is important because blood-sugar drops are directly related to hanger. To ward off hanger, keeping blood sugar stable is the goal. And researchers also found that participants who had the bar reported significantly greater pleasure in the class than those who drank only water. In other words, the dancers who ate breakfast enjoyed what they were doing more —

likely because they had more energy and were able to focus better.

You might not be dancing in a studio during the day. But you are dancing through your life. Sometimes it is very fast-paced and you may feel like you are twirling this way and that. But no matter the tune, you will take more pleasure in it and be able to be more mindfully present if you've had breakfast.

Keep in mind that breakfast doesn't have to be the traditional bacon and eggs or bowl of cereal. When I travel to Europe, I am often reminded that breakfast looks different to everyone. In the morning, Europeans often eat things Americans might eat for lunch, like an array of sliced meats and cheese. Protein like this is a great start for the day. In Japan, people often begin the day with a bowl of rice.

I tell my clients to let go of their idea of what they think breakfast "should" look like and start thinking about what works for them. What would you like to eat in the morning? And when? Maybe breakfast doesn't work well for you first thing, when you roll out of bed. Perhaps it would work better for you a bit later, for a few minutes at your desk before you start your day.

No matter what you choose for breakfast or when or where it happens, being more mindful of your breakfast routine may be one of the most important factors in managing hanger. Not only does breakfast have a profound impact on the body, it also affects your mood and ability to function for the rest of the day.

Hangry to Happy

Mind your breakfast. Be mindful of how your body responds with and without breakfast. How do you feel in the mornings if you eat breakfast or skip it? How do you feel throughout the day?

Define breakfast. What does it mean to you? And what could it look like? What time? What place? Specify a goal. For example: "Eating before 10:00 a.m., at my kitchen table, before I leave my house."

What are your obstacles to breakfast? Begin by assessing what has been standing in the way of eating breakfast. *Why* you aren't hungry for breakfast is the bigger issue to solve.

If you "aren't a breakfast person," think outside the box. Breakfast doesn't have to be cereal. What would you actually *like* to eat? It could even be a bite of last night's leftovers. Or a bowl of soup. Whatever powers you up!

If you aren't hungry at breakfast, it's likely that you are eating very late at night or your body is slow to wake up. Your body sets its internal clock by sleep patterns and eating. If you aren't hungry when you get up, drink some warm water or tea first thing. This can help wake up your digestive system. The first thing you eat sends a signal to your body—it's almost as if it turns on the lights and opens your metabolism for business. It fires up all systems in your body. If you are staying up too late, maybe that is the real issue to tackle. Another issue might be eating too late in the evening.

If you don't have time, portable items can be key. A banana is easy to throw in your purse. Or a yogurt that you can eat at your desk. Or anything else that you think is delicious and that is also easy to carry, like a hard-boiled egg, bag of granola, some slices of lunch meat rolled around cheese, a protein bar, or a breakfast tortilla with peanut butter and apple chunks rolled up inside.

Cookies! I love making what I call breakfast cookies. They are mainly oats, and I mix in whatever else I feel like or have, such as nuts and cranberries. I put them in a container and they are so easy for my family to eat or take along. Everyone has time for a cookie!

HUNGER HYPNOTIZER #27: NIGHTTIME NIBBLING

" 'I stand in front of an open refrigerator door, looking for answers.' This is a quote I saw on social media. It really struck a chord with me. I do this. Particularly at night. I find that I pick and pick and pick at food at night, when really, I just need to go to bed."

After dinner...

a) I always snack at night.
b) I sometimes want a snack in the evening.
c) I try not to eat after dinner.
d) I generally don't eat late at night.

People snack at night for different reasons.

Sometimes they're genuinely hungry. One of my clients has a husband who's retired. He has dinner waiting for her the moment she walks in the door from work at five o'clock. Then, they walk around the high school track. By nine, she's really hungry and wants a little something. For her, the trick was to find a filling snack that honors her hunger but doesn't have too much sugar or caffeine that could stimulate her system and keep her up all night.

For other clients, eating at night is just a habit. Like my client Aubrey. She and her husband, Eric, like to watch TV together at night. After a full day's work, they are both exhausted, and it is the only time they regularly spend together. At eight o'clock almost on the dot, her husband would wander into the kitchen, get a snack, and bring back a plate for both of them. Often, she didn't even want anything. But it was such a sweet, thoughtful gesture from Eric that she went ahead and ate anyway. Their daily routine meant she often went to bed feeling regretfull. And she didn't know how to get them both out of the habit.

My anxious clients are probably the ones who struggle the most with night eating. They are often up late because they just can't fall asleep or stay asleep. As soon as the lights turn off, their brains turn on. They begin to worry about everything under the sun. When we dig deep into their night eating habits, they often realize that they're trying to find foods to help them get to sleep and quiet down the brain. For them, eating helps to quash or mute anxiety. They sometimes eat until they fall into a "food coma," their stomachs so full that they can feel only that.

Hangry to Happy

Go to bed. Believe it or not, the majority of my clients who eat at night are not really hungry. They are simply tired. Exhausted, in fact. So before you take a bite at night, ask yourself, "Am I just tired?" I know it sounds simplistic, but if you answered yes, try going to bed. You would be amazed at how many of my clients have turned around night eating by giving themselves permission to go to bed. Their head often resists and says, "But I should stay up and do laundry...or pay bills...or read...." But when they acknowledge that their body is maxed out and it's okay to call it a day, they hit the sack instead of eating—which in the long run makes them very happy. Ask yourself, how tired are you on a scale from 1 (wide awake) to 10 (almost asleep and can barely keep your eyes open)? If you are anywhere above a 5, it's worth considering going to sleep.

Try sleep-aid snacks. If you do genuinely feel hungry before bed, there are some snacks that have been shown to help people fall asleep fast. In one study, participants fell asleep faster—in only 17 minutes, on average—when they ate healthy snacks, lower in saturated fat and higher in protein than the meals they chose for themselves.[81] In contrast, it took an average of 29 minutes for participants to fall asleep after eating the less healthy food and drinks they picked for themselves. Many of the foods contain helpful sleep compounds, including tryptophan, which contributes to production of serotonin, the feel-good neurotransmitter; melatonin; magnesium; and calcium—all of which are known to have a calming effect and help people go to sleep.[82]

Tart Cherries. In two studies, adults with insomnia who drank 8 ounces (237 ml) of tart cherry juice twice a day for two weeks slept about an hour and a half longer and reported better sleep quality, compared to nights they did not drink the juice.[83]

Kiwifruit. In a four-week study, 24 adults consumed two kiwifruits one hour before going to bed each night. At the end of the study, participants fell asleep 42 percent more quickly than when they didn't eat anything before bedtime. Additionally, their ability to sleep through the night without waking improved by 5 percent, while their total sleep time increased by 13 percent.[84]

Oatmeal. Whole-grain oatmeal is mostly carbohydrates—which can help you to become drowsy. Also, oats contain stress-reducing B$_6$ as well as melatonin, another natural sleep aid. Try eating a small bowl at night before you go to bed!

Tryptophan Foods. Tryptophan (also called L-tryptophan) is an essential amino acid. It acts like a natural mood regulator and can help you sleep! If you struggle with sleep, try a food that is a good source of tryptophan, such as a banana, sunflower seeds, pistachios, cashews, almonds, tofu, cheese, red meat, chicken, turkey, fish, oats, beans, lentils, potatoes, or eggs.

These are just a few examples. Experiment to find out which foods help you count sheep faster!

HUNGER HYPNOTIZER #28: FOODS THAT TURN FROWNS UPSIDE DOWN

"When I eat healthier foods, I notice that my mood is so much better. It's not dramatic, like I break into song or anything. But I very much notice the absence of that overeating 'I regret-eating-that' feeling. I hate that feeling. But a really good banana that is ripe the perfect amount, spread with some almond butter, is just a great snack. I feel like I made a good choice for me—even that is cool."

As far as healthy foods go . . .

a) I don't like healthy foods or how they taste.
b) I like healthy foods once in a while.
c) I eat a variety of foods—some healthy, some not.
d) There are a lot of healthy foods that make me happy.

Think for a moment about the last food you ate that made you unhappy. Maybe it wasn't the food itself but how it made you feel. Were you regretfull, too full, bloated? Did you get hungry again immediately, or too sugared up?

Most of us are well aware of which foods leave us feeling unhappy. My clients talk a lot about how heavy, fatty, fried, or sugary foods make them feel bad if they don't eat them mindfully. "I love BBQ chips," one of my clients told me. "But I always eat way too many of them and then feel just awful." And he's not alone. Many of my clients focus a lot on how terrible mindlessly eating certain foods can make them feel.

Now answer the flip side of that question. What food have you eaten recently that made you happy? Personally, I love mangoes. I don't buy them every single time I go to the store because they are expensive and not always in season. But I buy a lot of things that have mango in them, like mango smoothies and mango flavored tea, and I always jump at the chance to have one. For me, mangoes hit all the right sensory pleasure buttons. I also know that they are packed with vitamin C, and I feel good when I know I'm doing something good for my body. There's not much I like better than a perfectly ripe mango, from the sweet taste to the great smell.

When I go to the grocery store, my kids ask me to buy the "happy fruit." I know what they are talking about. The container has a logo on it of a kiwi with a happy smile. However, my kids didn't give kiwi its nickname because of the jolly little mascot. It's because I told them about an interesting study about kiwis, published in the *Journal of Nutritional Science*.[85] Researchers recruited 139 male students, 18 to 35 years old, to examine the impact of eating kiwifruit on mood. After researchers gave them a battery of tests on mood, the researchers discovered there was an inverse association of vitamin C levels with depression, confusion, and anger. In other words, those who ate the most fruit had the fewest problems with their mood.

In a previous study by this same author, just giving men two kiwis a day boosted young men's moods. Those who had the daily kiwi noted a decrease in fatigue, an increase in energy, and a trend toward a decrease in depression: a powerful confirmation that food can have a big impact on mood.

In the Hanger Management program, I ask my clients to shift their focus away from how some foods make them feel bad and instead toward noticing how some foods make them feel good—how some foods positively influence their mood. Often, they start out thinking that healthy foods don't affect them much: "I don't feel anything when I eat an apple." But when they start to pay attention, they begin to see this absence of feeling as a positive.

It's a little like if you were to twist your ankle. You don't usually appreciate how wonderful it is to walk around pain-free. But if you've suffered a big injury, the absence of pain is a delight. When my clients start tuning in to how foods make their body feel—relaxed, content, pleasant—it's the same thing. They start to tune in to the positives that are often overshadowed by the negative.

A study in *Frontiers in Psychology* looked at what specific foods often help people to be happier.[86] In particular, they looked at how both raw and processed fruits and vegetables influence depressive symptoms, anxiety, negative mood, positive mood, life satisfaction, and flourishing, among young adults in both the United States and New Zealand. Does eating fruits and vegetables help our mood? According to both this study and the many firsthand reports of my clients: Yes!

Hangry to Happy

Would you like to perk up your mood with healthy foods? My ten-day Hangry-to-Happy Challenge incorporates the top ten raw foods (in no particular order) that, according to that study, had the best effect on mental health. The great news: these foods don't require any cooking—just eat! I've made some suggestions for how to turn these raw foods into great snacks. But feel free to do whatever works for you.

10-Day Hangry-to-Happy Challenge. Each morning, rate your mood, from 1 to 10. And each day, eat one of the foods listed below. At the end of the day, rate your mood again.

Carrots. Dip them in dressing or hummus, or spread with almond or peanut butter and sprinkle cinnamon on top. Arrange in a flower by spreading baby carrots around a center ramekin. Roast into carrot fries. Bake slices into chips.

Bananas. Add Nutella or peanut butter; put on cereal; mash with avocado; blend into a smoothie. Freeze for a frozen confection. Layer between crackers. Make into energy balls or muffins.

Apples. Sprinkle with cinnamon or granola; spread with nut butter or cream cheese. Cut in half and make into a sandwich. Make applesauce or apple butter. Bake to make apple chips. Dice and put on yogurt, cottage cheese, ice cream, or toast. Layer with slices of sharp cheddar or Swiss cheese. Drizzle with caramel, honey, or dark chocolate.

Dark Leafy Greens (like spinach, kale, or swiss chard). Fill a salad bowl; put in soup, layer on sandwiches; or use as garnish for your plate. Add to breakfast items like eggs. Include in wraps. Use as pizza topping. Add to pasta. Tuck into tacos or use on baked potatoes. Use them as wraps. Bake into chips.

Grapefruit. Sprinkle with sugar (white or brown) or salt. Grill; blend into smoothies; drop into drinks. Garnish a salad. Add vanilla, honey, and yogurt. Make a grapefruit salsa. Drink grapefruit juice. Put on ice cream.

Lettuce. Use as a wrap instead of bread. Chop and put in soup. Grill. Top it like a cracker. Make it a filling in spring rolls, wraps, or tacos.

Other Citrus Fruits (like oranges, mandarin oranges, lemons, limes, and pomegranates). Put them in water. Sprinkle them in salads. Grill them with meat. Top a dessert like cheesecake with them.

Fresh Berries. Add to overnight oats; put in salads; serve with ice cream as a dessert. Blend into smoothies; make into salsa. Freeze and drop into drinking water; mix into muffins. Freeze into ice cubes. Make into fruit spread or jam.

Cucumber. Make into salad or tabouli. Add to pasta. Stuff into pita. Top it like a cracker; scoop into a dip like salsa or hummus. Make into a chunky salad. Skewer with fruit. Top with cheese.

Kiwifruit. Blend into smoothies; add to salad; use as a garnish. Put on toast or crackers. Chop into parfait. Use in salsa. Top with cinnamon or nutmeg.

HUNGER HYPNOTIZER #29: EAT BETTER, THINK BETTER

"My friends call me the snacking queen. I take snacks everywhere. I never leave home without them because I am a distracted hot mess who can hardly find her way home if I'm too hungry. I tried for a long time to give up snacking. But that really didn't work for me. Now I pack my bag with snacks. If I'm hungry, I pull out a bag of pistachios, and it's all better. When I didn't do this, I was at the mercy of the vending machine. I would eat whatever I could find to get my head on straight again."

If I'm feeling hungry...

a) I am often very distracted and can't think clearly at all.
b) thoughts about food interrupt what I'm doing.
c) my focus isn't as good as it is when I am well fed.
d) I don't have any problems focusing.

Hanger isn't just about being irritable. For many people, it shows up most prominently in how it decreases their ability to think clearly.

My clients will often come in rubbing their heads in utter dismay: "I just couldn't get anything done. I gave up working on the project because it was pointless unless I got something to eat. I was going in circles."

I experience food-related changes in my concentration level in my own life. I sit for eight hours a day straight, listening intently to people. I have to be able to concentrate. My mind can't wander for a second, or I might miss an important detail. So I have to bring snacks. Every day I pack up my bag for work: phone charger, keys, to-do list, and, most important, snacks.

Nothing's more frustrating than not being able to get things done when they need to be done. And sometimes the only thing that stands in the way of being productive is having a good meal or snack.

Ever wished you could take a magic pill that would make you smarter and better at your work? It may just be that apple sitting on your desk.

In one study, researchers had healthy participants eat the equivalent of a chocolate bar—48 grams of dark chocolate (70 percent cacao, with organic cane sugar). Then their brains were scanned with an EEG, which measures brain waves, 30 minutes and 60 minutes after eating. Gamma waves increased across multiple areas of the cortex, mainly related to cognition and memory.[87] The changes were most pronounced after 30 minutes and returned to normal by the 60-minute mark. In other words, eating dark chocolate helped people remember and make decisions.

Another study found that students who ate bananas before an exam did better than those who didn't, perhaps because bananas provide potassium, an essential mineral crucial for keeping your brain, nerves, and heart in tip-top shape. And a report published by the *Journal of Agricultural and Food Chemistry* showed that people who drank blueberry juice every day for two months significantly improved their performance on learning and memory tests.[88] But it doesn't have to be blueberry juice. For example, a study of schoolchildren showed that eating 1½ cups of fresh blueberries can provide important cognitive benefits, including improved reaction time and better short memory recall on tests.[89]

The take-home message: when we snack and eat foods mindfully, we have more focus, and we're better at our job—and our lives.

Hangry to Happy

Need a focus fix? Quickly assess how much focus and concentration you need today. Do you have to be completely on your game and paying attention to every single detail—because you're doing surgery, taking a test, or counting money? Or perhaps it's Saturday and you are going to veg out in front of the TV. You don't need or want to focus on anything! Hanger comes when there is a mismatch between how much focus you need and the food fuel you have given your brain. Nothing is more frustrating than being unable to concentrate!

Begin to tune in to your own concentration level throughout the day. Notice how it changes with different tasks, the time of day, your interest level in a project, distractions—and hunger level. What is your concentration level right now?

Make a snack tradition around concentration lags. I've learned some lessons about snacking while traveling to other countries. In France, I was introduced to a *goûter*, an eating occasion between lunch and dinner. The English have afternoon tea. *Merienda* (sometimes spelled *marenda* or *merenda*) is eaten in Spain, Portugal, Italy, Slovenia, Croatia, Hispanic America, and the Philippines. It is a small meal between lunch and dinner. All over the world, snacking is a tradition and custom. It's an accepted part of daily life.

Observe your daily routine and create your own snacking tradition. When do you struggle most with concentration? Morning? Afternoon? Many people experience a lull in their energy level around 3:00. Find a time during the day when you need more concentration—and plan to have a snack. And give your snack time a name, like "Focus Fuel."

Foods that help concentration. When it comes to concentration, some foods help more than others—a lot more.

Below is a list of foods that naturally boost concentration—and how they can help you.

Chocolate! Have some dark chocolate or a cup of cocoa! A study in the journal *Neurology* concluded that those who drank two cups of cocoa every day for a month had improved blood flow to the brain and performed better on memory tests.[90] And in another study, people who ate 48 grams of 70 percent cacao chocolate (1.5 ounces, or about two square inches) saw an improvement in brain functioning thirty minutes after consuming it.[91]

Omega-3. People who have high levels of omega-3s, healthy fatty acids found in fish, soybeans, and walnuts, show increased blood flow in the brain and better cognition, or thinking abilities.

Berries. A review of the benefits of berries (including strawberries, blackberries, blueberries, and blackcurrants) found great benefits to the brain. In particular, berries improve communication between brain cells. And they make a great "fuel-up" finger food.[92]

Vitamin E–rich Foods. Sunflower seeds, almonds, hazelnuts, mangoes, avocados, butternut squash, spinach, kiwis, broccoli, and tomatoes also help you think better. Vitamin E has antioxidant properties that protect your cells from stress and aging.

Beets and Beet Juice. These increase blood flow to the brain, helping concentration. In one study, forty healthy adults received either a placebo or 450 milliliters of beet-root juice during a ninety-minute period, then were given a series of tests. The result? Their cognitive performance was improved on simple subtraction, as well as other tasks. These results show that even a single dose of beet juice can help you think better.[93]

Foods with Natural Nitrites. Found in high concentrations in celery, cabbage, spinach, and other leafy green vegetables, nitrites are known to widen blood vessels. And researchers have recently discovered that nitrites also increase blood flow to the brain, boosting its performance.[94, 95]

Vitamin K–rich Foods. Foods rich in vitamin K include kale, edamame, pickles, broccoli, asparagus, pumpkin seeds, pine nuts, and blueberries. They help visual memory and verbal fluency. In other words, vitamin K helps us remember what we see and speak easily and clearly.[96]

Green Tea. It has been shown to be great for sharpening memory and attention.[97] Try some when you need to boost your powers of concentration!

HUNGER HYPNOTIZER #30: FOODS FOR ALL-DAY ENERGY

"By 3:00 in the afternoon, I could lay my head on my keyboard and fall fast asleep. I think to myself, 'Oh my gosh, I have got to wake up. I am never going to make it through the day.' But I can't drink coffee past noon because there is no way I will sleep at night. So a candy bar seems like a great option to help me power through until 5:00."

When I'm feeling low energy...

a) I eat sugary snacks for an energy boost.
b) I eat anything near me for some fuel.

c) I sometimes choose healthy foods to give me a boost.

d) I generally choose snacks that improve my energy levels.

We live in a word that is full of energy-sucking vampires — from toxic people to busy schedules to constantly being plugged into one's phone. Almost everyone feels tapped out at some point.

For me personally, most tasks without human-related interaction completely zap me of energy. Things like paperwork. Bills. Insurance papers. Filing.

What drains you of your energy the most? This is important to specify: exactly what tugs down your energy level. Because that's when hanger can pounce.

People who are dragging through their day for whatever reason often turn to what I call energy-drained eating. They have the right idea, basically. They know food can help fuel them up when they're low on energy. But the foods they choose can either help their mood — or drag them further down, into hanger.

One of my jobs in Hanger Management is to help people to think through what are they snacking on and how it is working for them. First, I ask them to tune into *why* they are snacking. Are they trying to get more energy? Trying to forget they're tired? Searching to find a bit of pleasure in the midst of an otherwise dreary day?

The clients in my virtual practice who often think the most about how food relates to energy level are teens involved in organized sports or adults who spend a lot of time playing a sport. Cory, a forty-five-year-old mom who plays tennis twice a week in a league, is a good example. She noticed that how she talks about and chooses food is very different from the ways a lot of other moms do. "I'm not interested in dieting or starving myself to be skinny," she told me. "I take my tennis league really seriously. The tennis league is the only thing that helps to curb my competitive edge. I google things like high-protein foods and foods that help me play way better. And I really like to win!"

People involved in sports and physical activities get the idea that food truly is fuel. It's often because they can see a very direct correlation between what they eat and how they perform. When they eat better, they can run the same exact distance much faster. They get really tangible results that others often can't see day to day. And that's convincing. I don't get a timer out to see how long it takes me to do paperwork. But I have noticed that I can get my notes done, shut off my computer, and be out the door within an hour after seeing patients—*if I am well fed and focused.* If not, it's easy to get distracted and have to finish up my paperwork the next day.

The good news is, lots of foods help to maintain energy and endurance. For example, a recent study showed that eating a banana prior to a 75 km cycling trial was just as effective as consuming a carbohydrate drink for improving the performance of endurance athletes.[98]

And in a small trial, participants who ate a dark-chocolate bar (but not a milk-chocolate bar) had significantly improved contrast sensitivity and visual acuity for two hours after eating it. Not only that, dark chocolate helped people to feel more satisfied.[99]

And this is where we have the opportunity to turn hangry into happy.

Hangry to Happy

Mind your energy need. One of the first things you need to do to prevent hanger is identify how much energy you need. Hanger happens when there's a mismatch between the energy we expend and what we eat to power ourselves. When we expend more energy than we consume, we run out of gas and get grumpy. So do a quick assessment in the morning as soon as you get up. What energy does your day require? Will you be moving a lot, working in the garden all day? Or do you plan to sit at your desk for eight hours? High-energy days require more fuel to keep you happy, not hangry!

Make a snack menu. Snacking is one of the best ways to prevent hanger. But my clients are often caught off guard by hanger, without a snack. It's helpful to have your snack options ready ahead of time, so you don't need to take time to think them through when you're already hungry. Consider how often and how comfortable we are consulting menus. So create your own! Stick a snack menu near your desk or on your fridge, or put it on a chalkboard. List at least three snack options, covering common snacking desires—salty, sweet, and savory options. When you need one, you won't even have to think too hard—just choose from your predetermined menu. Be sure to stock up on these snacks and any ingredients you need for them.

Eat energy-boosting foods. Energy-boosting snacks provide fuel for your body, and that fuel can come in many forms: apple slices with peanut butter, popcorn sprinkled with spices or cheese, cheese kabobs, spicy chickpeas, almonds, hard-boiled eggs, energy bites, pumpkin seeds, dark-chocolate squares. Apples have a high antioxidant content, and research has shown that antioxidants may slow down the digestion of carbohydrates, so energy is released over an extended period of time. Bananas are great for fueling up because they are an excellent source of carbohydrates, potassium, and vitamin B_6, all of which can help boost energy levels in your body. And yogurt contains sugars that can provide ready-to-use energy.

Remember: these are just ideas. Everyone's different, and what you need may be different from what anyone else needs.

You need to find what provides YOU with sustained energy. What is most important is that your snacks provide the right kind of fuel to power your day—whatever it may bring you.

Make custom trail mixes. Creating your own blend of trail mix can be the best of all worlds. You can put together all kinds of things, as long as they include a lot of nutrients to benefit your mood and reduce your hanger level. Choose any combination that sounds good to you: chocolate or yogurt bites; dried fruit such as bananas, apricots, or cherries; cranberries; goji berries; pumpkin seeds; sunflower seeds; M&M's; peanut butter chips; popcorn; nuts; coconut flakes; coffee or espresso beans; oatmeal; granola; cereal; sesame sticks. Enhance your mix with Cajun seasoning, sea salt, or cinnamon. Then put the mix in a baggie and carry it with you for an energy boost.

Stash emergency hanger snack kits. This is one of the best tricks my clients have learned, to keep them from grabbing the first thing within arm's reach. Think of it like the other emergency items you may have in your bag—a Band-Aid or extra cash. And choose things that can stay fresh in your bag until you need them.

HUNGER HYPNOTIZER #31: THE BALANCING ACT

"Whenever I feel overwhelmed, all I crave are highly processed carbs and comfort foods—like bagels, sugar cereals, and cookies. But eating them makes me sleepy. So I started making sure that I had more balance whenever I eat. If I eat a piece of bread, I put a piece of cheese on top, for exam-

ple. Making sure I don't drown myself in comfort food completely helps my mood."

When it comes to eating . . .

a) I find myself craving carbohydrates.
b) I like a lot of carbs but eat other foods.
c) I eat some different kinds of food.
d) I intentionally eat a diversity of foods.

My clients talk a lot about desperately craving carbohydrate-rich comfort foods such as donuts, muffins, pasta, mac and cheese, cake, and cookies, particularly when they are stressed or hangry. This makes sense. Carbohydrates are a quick way to get a dopamine hit and release serotonin, a feel-good chemical, in the brain.

What my clients learn over time is that when anything is out of balance in what we eat, it can lead to hanger. If we're overdosing on or craving just one type of food, whether it is carbohydrates or fatty fast food, it should give us pause. In fact, take a pause right now to think about how any kind of imbalance might be contributing to your hanger level. Is there something that you eat significantly more of than any other food?

My clients tell me about their good times with food—like how delighted they were to discover a spicy shrimp appetizer at the Thai bistro down the street. And they talk about the bad times, like the guilt they experienced when they ate an entire pepperoni pizza on their own, no sharing. But they don't just talk about their emotional response. They also talk about how different foods affect their hunger levels. Some foods leave them feeling hungry, seemingly no matter how much they gobble. But others leave them feeling satisfied all afternoon.

When we take a close look at what they are eating that leads to hanger, we often find that they are the most unsatisfied when their food choices are out of balance.

Sandy, a forty-seven-year-old single mom, worked as a teacher in a public school. Her job was stressful—managing a class full of hormonal middle schoolers. And teaching required her to be on her feet all day long, with very little time for herself. She had barely any time to use the bathroom and only a few moments between classes for snacks or lunch.

When she started working on her Hanger Management, she noticed that all she was eating during the day were carbohydrate-rich foods that were easy to eat as students streamed in and out between classes, such as pretzels, cookies, and muffins. "All I ate for days was carbohydrates," she told me. "I almost put myself into a carbohydrate coma each day."

For Sandy, all the pieces really began to fall into place one day when she ran out of her standard bagels at home. The bagels she was used to eating were huge, so she'd assumed that they'd keep her feeling full through her hectic mornings. But when she ran out of bagels, she grabbed some eggs from her fridge, scrambled them, and topped them with cheese. And even though it didn't seem like as much food as her giant bagel, she found she was much less hungry throughout the day.

She began to notice how different types of food affected her mood. So one day, after starting the Hanger Management program, Sandy decided to switch things up. She brought a baggie full of almonds with her to school.

"When I ate the almonds," she said, "I noticed a huge difference in my hanger level. And my students did, too. I wasn't irritable by the end of class, giving them my raised, stern teacher voice. The almonds tackled my hunger amazingly, in a way that a muffin couldn't even touch." (And this is no surprise, as almonds have been shown to help people feel more satiated.)[100]

The secret, for Sandy and for many of my other clients, was making sure she wasn't stuck on a one-way track, eating only carbohydrates. To remedy this, Sandy didn't stop eating carbohydrates, which she loves. Instead, she added protein-rich foods like eggs, almonds, and cheese during the day.

Sandy's strategy was based on good science, because study after study links protein with higher levels of feeling satisfied — exactly what she needed!

In one study, researchers asked subjects to eat two different yogurt snacks in the afternoon. The snacks were similar — except that one group of the participants had a high-protein yogurt, and some had a low-protein yogurt. The result? The people who ate the high-protein snack were less hungry and ate less later than those who didn't get as much protein.[101]

Another study found that eating eggs for breakfast, rather than a bagel, increased fullness and led to less calorie intake over the next thirty-six hours.[102] And yet another study found that a protein-rich breakfast of eggs and lean beef increased fullness and helped people make more mindful food choices throughout the day.[103]

In this tip, I've talked about carbohydrates being out of balance, because carbohydrates are what my clients who stress eat talk about craving the most. And they also talk about how much their mood and satisfaction level benefit when they balance carbohydrates with other foods. But carbohydrates aren't the only culprit — you could be overloading on any type of food.

Hangry to Happy

Balance check. For a moment, think about whether your food choices are out of balance in any way. Do you seek out one type of food above the others when stressed or hangry—carbohydrates, sugar, fruit, fast food? If so, how does relying so heavily on these foods affect your mood? Does it make you feel tired? Guilty? Bored? Something else?

Your hanger balance challenge: To maintain a good mood, intentionally add some balance whenever you eat. Maybe you pair a piece of chocolate with a piece of fruit. Or wrap a piece of meat in a tortilla. Put a piece of cheese on a cracker. If you eat mainly sweet snacks, pair them with something savory. Adding a contrasting food helps ensure you are getting all your nutrient needs covered, to help maintain your mood. If you eat a fast food, balance it with something homemade.

If you are someone who craves carbohydrates, remember, that is okay! Try an experiment in managing your hanger by adding more protein. As discussed above, people feel fuller and therefore happier when they have enough protein in their diet. So include foods containing protein in each meal. Some good options:

- chicken
- turkey
- beef
- fish
- eggs
- milk
- cheese
- yogurt
- oats
- soybeans
- chickpeas
- lentils

- broccoli
- spinach
- Brussels sprouts
- almonds
- peanuts

After you eat protein, write down how hungry you are on a scale of 1 to 10.

Then keep track of how long it takes you to get hungry after you eat protein: Three minutes? Thirty minutes? Three hours?

And keep asking yourself, "Do I feel hangry or happy when my food choices are more balanced?"

HUNGER HYPNOTIZER #32: DRINK UP!

"I used to get a lot of headaches and felt low energy—which made me pretty grumpy and hangry. Now, I do two things that help a lot. I carry a water bottle everywhere. And I eat a lot of foods that have a lot of water in them. Watermelon is my favorite—92 percent water."

When it comes to water...

a) I don't drink enough.
b) I hate it. It's so boring and bland.
c) I drink water with meals if it is served to me.
d) I make an active effort to hydrate. I carry a water bottle with me all day long.

Imagine for a moment that you are at a restaurant.

"Would you like a glass of water?" the waiter asks.

Do you say yes or no?

And if you say yes, do you actually drink it?

This is a pretty typical scenario at just about any American restaurant. We often take for granted the fact that water is free, readily available, and routinely offered or provided at the beginning of meals at American restaurants.

But in other countries, it's not.

One of my clients realized this on a recent trip to Sicily. In Sicily, a glass of water with a meal isn't free. And it's not free in many other places in the world. At every meal, she had to buy water and decide whether she wanted it "still" or "with bubbles." The charge for water is due to many factors, such as higher cost associated with water, filtration, and simply building in a fee for service.

That trip helped shift my client's mindset about drinking water. When she had to pay for water at a restaurant, my client suddenly became conscious of the role water plays in her meals. She craved it. She thought about how thirsty she was. She became aware of how not having water makes her feel. And how refreshing a glass is before a meal.

Even though American restaurants routinely serve water with meals, only a small percentage of people do the same at home. The good news is that water is one of the best tools we have for managing hanger.

Research has shown this time and again. For example, researchers from the University of Birmingham showed that drinking 16.9 ounces, or about one tall glass of water, before every meal can help to manage your appetite.[104] In this study, 84 adults were invited to participate in a twelve-week program. They all received advice on improving their diet and physical activity.

Then they were put into two groups. The first group was instructed to drink 16.9 ounces of water thirty minutes before their three daily meals every day for twelve weeks. The second, a control group, was told to imagine having a full stomach before every meal without drinking any water. This was just to make the subjects think that they were receiving an intervention.

The result?

Those in the group who were instructed to "preload" with water lost, on average, 1.3 kilograms (2.87 pounds), while those in the control group lost only 0.8 kilograms (or 1.76 pounds).

The bottom line: when you are trying to manage your appetite and eat more mindfully, staying hydrated is key.

Hangry to Happy

To help my clients make water work for them, I often tell them to start increasing the amount of water they drink every day. It's one of the easiest changes you can make to curb your hunger.

Hanger hydrating food challenge: Add at least one hydrating food every day, such as watermelon, strawberries, cantaloupe, peaches, oranges, skim milk, cucumbers, lettuce, zucchini, grapes, celery, yogurt, tomatoes, bell peppers, grapefruit, or coconut water. One of my favorites is frozen grapes! Think of it as an experiment, and take note of how adding these foods affects your mood and appetite.

Drink when you eat. Drink water before mealtimes. How much, and how close to a meal? Research shows that drinking 568 milliliters of water (about 2.4 cups) thirty minutes before a meal is ideal to help you to eat more mindfully at the next meal. Compared to those who did not drink water before a meal, pre-meal water drinkers reported increased fullness, satisfaction, and decreased hunger after the meal.[105] So pretend your dining table is a restaurant, and take some time to have a drink before your meal arrives. Studies show that people who drink two glasses of water immediately before a meal eat 22 percent less than those who don't drink any water.[106] But remember: Hanger Management is not about eating less, it's about being more mindful.

Start with soup. Because soup is high in liquid content, starting your meal with soup may also help manage your appetite. Researchers have observed that eating a bowl of soup at the beginning of a meal decreased hunger and reduced total calorie intake from the meal by about 100 calories.[107]

Set a specific goal. Observe your hydration habits to get a baseline of how much water you typically take in. Then increase your daily intake by half a cup at a time, or whatever amount you can manage. Knowing your goal helps you hit what you're aiming for. If you tend to forget, phone hydration apps can help. Go right now. Get a glass of water and give it a try!

Set deadlines and reminders. Set alarms to remind you to take a drink! Or set a deadline: "I will drink a glass of water by 10:00 a.m."

Keep cold water handy. Stash it in a jug in your fridge to have on hand at a moment's notice. If you don't like plain-Jane water, add sliced limes or lemons to make it more flavorful.

Connect hydration with established routines. When it's hard to remember a new behavior or routine, it's helpful to link it with one that is already first set in place. For example, you probably brush your teeth twice a day without any thinking or effort. So drink a glass of water after you brush. Easy!

HUNGER HYPNOTIZER #33: MOOD-BOOSTING VITAMIN D

"I have struggled a lot with feeling tired and down, and using emotional eating to cope. I feel a lot of guilt and self-blame for feeling this way when there is nothing wrong in my life besides ordinary daily stressors. I was shocked when my doctor indicated that feeling blue might be related to my diet. My vitamin D level was off the charts low. Getting my vitamin D level back on track made a phenomenal difference to how I feel and eat. It helped me put the brakes on my stress eating."

When it comes to vitamin D . . .

a) I have no idea if I get any.
b) I don't eat a lot of fatty fish, dairy, or eggs, so I doubt I get much vitamin D. I also don't spend much time out in the sun, which is where people often get it.
c) I try to eat a diverse diet and exercise outdoors, so it's likely I have enough vitamin D.
d) I often eat vitamin D–rich foods and have had my vitamin D level tested.

When Melanie was struggling with overeating, particularly emotional eating, one of the first things I recommended was to ask her doctor to have her blood work evaluated. Hormone, vitamin, and mineral levels can all influence your mood and hunger level. And Melanie was surprised when she found she was very low in vitamin D.

The signs that you might be low on vitamin D are all the kinds of things we often brush off or chalk up to other causes: depression, bone issues, exhaustion, muscle fatigue, weight gain, and issues with mood. It's easy to tell ourselves we must be upset or tired because of something besides a vitamin deficiency. And it's hard to keep track of our vitamin D levels because we can't see them without running a test.

Time and again, my clients who struggle with hanger and feeling regretfull turn out to have a low vitamin D level. And they're not alone. Almost three out of every four people in the world are low on vitamin D.[108]

What does vitamin D have to do with reducing hanger? A lot! Multiple studies have shown that people who are overweight are low in vitamin D levels.[109] But why? One theory says that vitamin D helps your brain produce serotonin, which increases feelings of happiness. Scientists have found that people with low vitamin D have a higher incidence of depression than those with normal levels.[110] And when you're feeling blue, you are much more likely to turn to food for comfort or to change your mood.

But vitamin D doesn't just affect our mood. It also improves strategic and analytic thought, planning, and decision-making. So getting enough vitamin D can also help us think through our food choices more mindfully.[111]

Hangry to Happy

Talk to your doc. If you struggle with appetite, emotional eating, and hanger, you may want to talk to your doctor about your vitamin D level and have it checked.

Let the sunshine in. The best way to get vitamin D is also easy: from sunlight between 10:00 a.m. and 3:00 p.m. Spend five to thirty minutes outside a few times a week. A light box (easily found online) can also help you soak up vitamin D from the rays when you're unable to get outside.

Try a supplement. In one study, clients who added vitamin

D supplements lost nearly twelve pounds and 5.48 cm around the waist.[112] And while vitamin D is well tolerated at doses higher than the recommended daily allowance, it is best to know how much YOU need. To find this out, talk with your doctor.

Vitamin D hanger challenge. Boost your vitamin D and see if it has an impact on your hanger level. Try to add one vitamin D–rich food every day, such as fatty fish like tuna and salmon, milk, vitamin D–fortified soy milk or orange juice, some cereals, Swiss cheese, and egg yolks, and note the impact on your mood and hanger level. Mushrooms grown outdoors naturally create vitamin D components from sunlight. If you love mushrooms, be sure to try chanterelles, maitake, and morels.

Bright and early. What's a particularly good time to consume vitamin D? You may find it easiest to weave vitamin D into breakfast. Almost all milk sold in the United States is fortified with vitamin D, and a growing number of food manufacturers are fortifying breakfast cereal, yogurt, margarine, and orange juice. For example, a cup of fortified orange juice contains 100 IU of vitamin D. People who eat breakfast have been found to have better levels of vitamin D than those who skip breakfast.[113] According to studies, consuming vitamin D positively affects serotonin levels, which helps you feel good.[114] Also, every tissue in the body has vitamin D receptors: every part of you needs vitamin D to function well.

HUNGER HYPNOTIZER #34: MOOD-BOOSTING MAGNESIUM

"My metabolism is very, very slow and I have cravings all the time. My doctor asked if I was getting enough magnesium in my diet. She said it could have an effect on my anxiety, not just my cravings. I had no idea what magnesium had to do with my body or what it did."

As far as my worry level...

a) I have a lot of anxiety.
b) I have mild anxiety.
c) I only worry about important things.
d) I don't worry much.

Each session, my client Jessica shares all the things that set her heart off beating faster and leave her feeling restless. She knows she struggles with anxiety, and she could come up with a never-ending list of worries, from *Will it rain tomorrow?* to *Will I get Alzheimer's when I am old?* It doesn't take much to trigger her anxiety. But Jessica notices it most when she is traveling for work or otherwise out of her normal routine or when a change that she can't control comes up.

Jessica and I work together on ways to calm her fight-or-flight system. And one of the tools we use is to increase how many magnesium-rich foods she eats.

If you worry a lot or struggle with feeling anxious, magnesium-rich foods may be a key to help to reduce your hanger. It's important to be mindful of your body and what it is telling you. Sometimes, your body is trying to tell you that some wires are getting crossed. And magnesium may help you untangle these wires. It's the fourth most abundant mineral in your body. It is part of over 300 of the chemical reactions that power and heal you.

Foods rich in magnesium have also been linked with reduced anxiety levels.[115] And magnesium is found in many foods. But it's virtually nonexistent in processed and fried foods, which is why many people, like Jessica, have a magnesium deficit. Approximately two thirds of individuals in the Western world have low magnesium levels.[116]

Magnesium-filled foods aren't a magic wand. But when Jessica began to introduce foods with magnesium into her diet, she noticed that her anxiety level seemed to be a notch lower. And that helped her to think more clearly, make better decisions—and also just relax every now and then. It was huge triumph, she told me, when she was able to sit and watch a few minutes of TV without needing to have something else in her hands or to hop up and down during a program. Instead, she just put her feet up and enjoyed the show.

Hangry to Happy

Hanger challenge: Magnesium week. Add some magnesium-rich foods to your diet for a week—at least one of these foods a day. Magnesium-rich foods include spinach, dark chocolate, tofu, whole grains, Swiss chard, black beans, almonds, cashews, potatoes, pumpkin seeds, avocados, bananas, broccoli, Brussels sprouts, flaxseeds, oatmeal, and carrots. At the end of the week, ask how you felt over the course of the week. Did you fret less? Feel calmer? Less hangry? Does it make sense to make magnesium a more permanent part of your diet? A good rule of thumb is that foods that have fiber often have magnesium in them.

> **Pumpkin Seeds.** One of my favorite magnesium-rich foods is pumpkin seeds. Studies show that eating 65 grams of pumpkin seeds reduces spikes in blood sugar following a meal—which makes it a great snack for turning hanger to happiness.[117]
>
> **Avocado.** Cut a slice of avocado and use it to top a sandwich or salad. Fill an avocado half with meat or veggies. Or mash the avocado like butter and spread it on toast. An interesting study looked at people who put a slice of avocado on a burger vs. those who did not. Turns out,

the avocado was helpful in reducing inflammation, which is often related to anxiety.[118] Yes! Just adding one slice of avocado to a hamburger made a difference!

Magnesium Body Butter. This is not the kind of butter you eat! You can absorb magnesium through your skin to your bloodstream with a cream. You can buy a jar of it or look up an online tutorial on how to make a magnesium-rich cream yourself. (Be sure your doctor says it's okay.)

HUNGER HYPNOTIZER #35: MOOD-BOOSTING CINNAMON

"Since my dietitian recommended that I increase my use of cinnamon on my food I have been carrying it around like it is a shaker of salt. It's a wonderful spice and I can sprinkle it on about anything—even things that I had not thought of—yogurt, in my coffee, on toast. In my eyes, it's a win-win. It tastes great and it helps to regulate my blood sugar and in turn makes me a happier, more even-keeled person."

When it comes to cinnamon...

a) I don't really like it.
b) I don't use cinnamon at all, unless it shows up in a recipe.
c) I like the smell of cinnamon and eat foods with cinnamon in them.
d) I love cinnamon and use it often.

I may be a doctor of psychology, but many of my clients are scientists in their own right—especially when it comes to experimenting on themselves.

And one of the things my diabetic clients study most closely is what happens when their blood sugar gets out of whack. I've learned a lot about how blood sugar affects mood by listening to them. And what they describe isn't pretty. Blood sugar has an immediate and serious impact on how people feel. No matter what else is going on, blood sugar that is too low or too high can completely overtake your emotions.

So many of my clients become experts on how to tell when their blood sugar is out of range. My client Julie, for example, tests her blood-sugar levels several times a day. And it was when she first started doing this that she began to recognize the connection between her emotions and her blood sugar. Seeing the numbers and comparing them to how she felt convinced her of the connection.

Now she's gotten so good at recognizing how she feels that she can usually guess her blood-sugar level correctly before she takes a test. "I started to feel really terrible. I feel irritable and worn out," she'll tell me. "So I tested my blood sugar, and I was absolutely right. It was way off."

And Julie isn't the only one who notices how blood sugar affects her. Before he saw the connection between her blood-sugar numbers and mood, Julie's husband thought she must just be moody, about all kinds of different things. Now, he'll sometimes say, "Is your blood-sugar level off? You just aren't yourself today. Do you want to check it?"

Remember: you don't need to have diabetes for your blood sugar to affect your mood. And one of the natural ways my clients have found to influence their blood sugar is through using cinnamon. This spice has been used for centuries in cultures around the world. And it doesn't just taste great. Some promising studies have shown that it offers health benefits;[119] for instance, it may lower blood-glucose levels in people with diabetes.[120] In one study, participants ate 1 to 6 grams of cinnamon for forty days and lowered their blood-sugar levels significantly.[121] So if you have trouble with high blood sugar, consider upping your cinnamon.

Keep in mind that more research is being conducted with cinnamon to understand how the different kinds of cinnamon affect people and whether it is helpful for everyone — some studies have not seen the same results. Some current studies are small and need to be replicated.

You can do your own experiments to see if cinnamon is a helpful tool for managing your hanger!

Hangry to Happy

Start small. Even a tiny amount of cinnamon can pack a big health punch. In a 2016 study, twenty-five people with poorly controlled diabetes consumed just 1g (a bit less than half a teaspoon) of cinnamon daily for twelve weeks and still reduced their fasting blood-sugar levels.[122] So add just a bit to your own diet — and be mindful of whether it has any effect on your mood.

Shake it up. Toss a shaker of cinnamon in your bag or purse. Easy access will make it more likely for you to reach for it.

Try cinnamon sticks. Buy some cinnamon sticks and use them as a spoon to stir your coffee, tea, yogurt, or soup. Or throw a whole stick in the pan while cooking meat or vegetables.

Change up coffee. Add cinnamon to your coffee or cocoa. A few sprinkles can boost the flavor, too!

Have a bit at breakfast. Start your morning with cinnamon: on oatmeal, granola, toast, yogurt, cereal, or whatever you like for breakfast.

Spice up fruit. Cinnamon is a great complement to berries and apples.

Important: Cinnamon is a natural way to help manage high blood sugar, but it contains a blood thinner and may have negative side effects, particularly for those on blood thinning medication. Also, do not use if you have liver damage. Consult your doctor to make sure it doesn't conflict with your medications or create health risks.

SUMMARY OF HUNGER HYPNOTIZERS

In this chapter, we drilled down on a specific point: what you eat doesn't just fill your belly. That's just one small, teeny-tiny part of it. What you eat also has an impact on whether you are happy today, how irritable you are, how you move, and how comfortable you feel in your skin.

From this day forward, you can become an expert at connecting the dots each day, between *this is what I ate* and *this is how I feel*.

I've mentioned a few themes that I hear my clients connect the dots for themselves. But there are so many more. And what we've talked about here is just a way to get you started.

So keep making your own connections by completing these sentences:

When I eat (fill in the blank) food, I feel...
When I eat (fill in the blank) food, I think...
When I eat (fill in the blank) food, I move...

And the checklist below can be a handy reference to connect the dots about opportunities in your life to hypnotize your own hunger.

___ I choose foods that keep me satisfied for a long period of time.
___ I eat foods at night that help me sleep.
___ I eat foods that help improve my mood.

___ I eat foods that help me think better.

___ I eat a balance of foods.

___ I drink enough water.

___ I make sure I get enough vitamin D.

___ I make sure I get enough magnesium.

___ I use cinnamon and spices to help manage taste and mood.

Hack Your Habits: 10 *S*'s of Mindful Eating

Think for a moment about the last thing that you ate mindfully: something you really enjoyed, and ate just the right amount of to feel very satisfied.

What was it?

For me, it was a peach. I ate it this morning. I could smell the peach from across the room. I pushed my computer to the side and stopped writing this passage. I cut up the peach, mindfully. It was sweet. And sticky. And delicious. Most important, I had no urge to eat while typing this. Two minutes with just the peach was worth taking a break from my work.

In a nutshell, mindful eating is being more aware of *how* you eat—from how you choose your food, to how you munch on it, to how it affects your mood and body. This sounds like a ridiculously simple definition. But for my clients, it's one of the most important skills that has helped them shed old habits and break out of their hanger cycle.

It takes some effort and attention for my clients to get the hang of mindful eating. But once they do, they don't go back. They almost can't. Because now they spot their mindless eating triggers and traps a mile away.

We often approach eating in a very routine, cookie-cutter way. We use the same approach over and over. We fall into the same habits. That's because our brain loves to operate on autopilot. It likes routine and easy behaviors. But many of our familiar habits lead us right to hungriness, day after day.

To do anything about that, first we have to *see* our habits. And that's easier said than done—even when you've been practicing mindfulness for a long time.

I've been eating mindfully for the past twenty years. But I still run across new mindless eating challenges all the time. For instance, I recently started eating lunch with one of my friends on a regular basis. We often eat lunch together on Fridays between meetings. We don't have long for lunch, and we want to have time to really connect. So without even realizing it, we started to eat really quickly. We didn't talk about it. It just happened. Then I started to notice that I didn't like how I felt after the first two lunches. So I called ahead and ordered our lunch so it was ready when we got there. That gave us an extra twenty minutes to eat—enough time to slow down and enjoy both lunch and our chat.

My newest mindful eating challenge isn't for myself. It's teaching my kids how to eat mindfully. I've been working with them on developing mindful eating since they were toddlers. They get the concept. But I can see the way other habits constantly try to override their mindful eating skills. The other day, one of my kids got a snack, then flipped on the TV and sat down at the table. I could see an "Oh, wait!" look cross his face. Then he got up and turned the TV off. It's not always easy to protect good habits—but it can be done.

Whatever new eating situation may pop up for you, mindful eating solutions always have one thing in common: being aware of how you eat and how you feel.

In this section, we will talk about the 10 S's of mindful eating: simple steps to help you change the *way* you eat. I developed them because my clients needed concrete tools for change, to move from hanger to happiness.

HACK YOUR HABITS #36: **S**ELECT, DON'T JUST EAT!

"A big step for me in learning to eat more mindfully was to stop my habit of responding immediately whenever my mind said 'I'm hungry.' What I found is that my mind actually tells me that a lot—like all the time. When I truly take a time-out and think it through, my next thought is sometimes 'Yes, I am hungry.' But about 40 percent of the time, the answer is, 'Not really.' This surprised me. I had never slowed down enough to pause or even question it."

When I choose what to eat . . .

a) I am paralyzed by indecision.
b) I eat the first thing that's available and convenient.
c) I identify a few options.
d) I consider my options carefully.

In the fourteenth century, the French philosopher Jean Buridan described a donkey that was unable to choose between two bales of hay. The story has a sad ending: eventually, the indecisive creature starved to death.

A lot of my clients have a conundrum like that donkey's: deciding what to eat and when to eat it. Thankfully, they don't starve to death. But indecision can be frustrating. And when we don't make conscious decisions, we often fall into habits and routines that we wind up regretting later.

How many times have you eaten a meal, then thought, "Darn, that wasn't what I really wanted"? Or "Why did I eat that?" Those are the post-eating regret blues. And they often come about because we didn't take the time to select our food in advance. We just ate whatever was there.

In my Hanger Management program, clients learn to eat mindfully, with intention. From the very start, they make decisions about what they want and why, so they don't find themselves eating something they didn't really want or need.

And want to guess what my clients like best about this stage of mindful eating? They love that the very first step is to do nothing. Instead of taking action—eating—they simply hold back and give themselves time to make a selection.

Hangry to Happy

When it's time for you to select your next snack or meal, just remember 3 *P*'s: Pause, Position, Pick.

Pause. When you think you're hungry—because your mind tells you that you want something or because there is food nearby—take a thirty-second PAUSE. My clients often say this word to themselves in their head. When they do, they realize that, before, they almost never put the brakes on their hunger or questioned it.

Position. According to the psychological theory of embodied cognition, pairing a thought with an action influences what you do.[123] If you pair a pause in your mind with an actual pause in your body language, you're more likely to take the break you need. So think of an action that will remind you to be more mindful. For instance: lift your foot off the ground, as if about to step on a brake pedal to slow down. Or make a stop signal with your hand. Or press your hand down onto the table, as if pushing an invisible pause button.

Pick. As you pause, ask yourself, "What would be a mindful choice in this moment?" The answer may be "Eat!" But it might also be something else, like "Take a nap!" Or take a break or switch tasks because you are bored. It might take something other than food to really satisfy you. A helpful rule of thumb when selecting food options is to limit your choices—three or fewer. We get very overwhelmed by too many choices. Think about a menu that is multiple pages, as opposed to a one-page menu.

HACK YOUR HABITS #37: **S**WITCH IT UP

"I love switching up my snacks. Otherwise I get bored with a food and sometimes 'OD' on it. It gets to the point that I begin to get sick of foods when I eat them too often."

When I eat...

a) I eat almost exactly the same foods every day.
b) I have a pretty set list of foods I eat and restaurants I go to.
c) I am a flexible eater.
d) I prefer adventure and new foods. I'll try anything.

Several years ago, I visited a friend in NYC. He bought two gigantic slices of pizza from a vendor on the street and handed me one. As I began to awkwardly take a bite, he said, "Whoa,

whoa, whoa! That is not how you eat a slice of pizza in New York City."

Then he folded his slice in half. I'm from the Midwest, where we never fold our pizza. In Chicago I'd tried deep dish, but with the help of a knife and fork. "But when in Rome—or New York," I thought, and copied my friend. Eating pizza is nothing new for me. But eating it that way completely changed the experience.

Over time, the things that give us pleasure start to give us less pleasure than they used to. Psychologists call this *hedonistic adaptation*. Things that once made us happy begin to lose their luster after we've done them repeatedly. It can happen with anything from a new car to a new relationship. And it happens with food, too.

Restaurants know this. That's why they advertise new gimmicks with food: eating standing up, or in the dark, or with no utensils. People flock to the new experience.

But does it work? In a recent study, researchers asked participants to eat popcorn. Half were asked to eat the popcorn the normal way, with their hands. The others were told to eat it with chopsticks. Those who ate with the chopsticks enjoyed the popcorn significantly more than others.[124]

In a second part of the study, 300 participants rated drinking water as more enjoyable when it was imbibed in new ways. In this research, participants came up with their own novel ideas for drinking water. They suggested everything from drinking out of a martini or wine glass to lapping the water out of a cup with their tongue like a cat. They all enjoyed drinking water more in these novel ways.

Why? Because when something is new, we pay more attention to it. And when we pay more attention to something, we enjoy it more.

Even foods we love, like ice cream and cookies, become boring over time. We stop savoring each bite with amazement. Foods that we eat routinely and that we like become familiar and mundane.

The bottom line is that when we eat *more* of something, we actually enjoy it *less*.

One of the simplest pieces of advice I give my clients might also sound just a little crazy: sit in a different spot at the kitchen table. Why? Because most people tend to sit in exactly the same seat when they eat. Simply sitting in a different spot can change the experience significantly.

If you want to enjoy your food more, the trick is to shake up your normal patterns. It's doing something different that will give you more pleasure—not more food.

Hangry to Happy

Find a new spot. Look for a new view or a new space to eat. It can be a different spot at the dining-room table or new seat in the break room. Or picnic on the floor or on your bed.

Use your fingers. In Ethiopian cuisine, for example, people use their hands rather than silverware to scoop up food, using bread. Using our fingers helps us to feel the texture and be more mindful of what we eat.

Unique combinations. Forget the ordinary. Sprinkle your favorite food, no matter what it is, with your favorite spice. Try cinnamon on chili, or salt on dessert!

Different glassware. Try drinking water out of a martini or wine glass, and add fruit garnishes to help your family members hydrate—particularly those who dislike plain water.

Experiment with utensils. Eat pizza with a knife and fork to slow you down. For ice cream, try a fork or baby spoon.

Switch hands. Eat with your non-dominant hand. If you're right-handed, hold your fork with your left hand instead of your right.

Eat backward. Eat the cupcake first, then the icing. Or eat your favorite food first instead of saving the best for last.

Freeze/heat foods. A change in temperature can change everything. Put grapes in the freezer or pop chocolate into the microwave to warm it up.

HACK YOUR HABITS #38: **S**IT: ALWAYS EAT OFF YOUR FEET

"I hate parties where there's food but no seats. I find myself trying to juggle my plate and talk. I like sitting down so I can enjoy my food. When I stand, I tend to munch without really thinking. Even worse, I stand beside the appetizer table and nibble away."

I most often eat...

a) leaning against the counter.
b) walking around the kitchen or office.
c) on the couch in front of the TV.
d) sitting at the kitchen table.

Recently, I went to New York City with my daughter. Our ritual is to buy a cupcake from one of the city's amazing bakeries and share it. On this particular day, we were in the West Village. We bought one vanilla cupcake with cookie dough icing. The woman put it in a clear plastic container for us to transport back to our hotel. I noticed my daughter eyeing it hungrily as we walked. When we got to Washington Square Park, she said, "How about if we sit down to eat, so we can enjoy it?"

It was a great mindful moment. Instead of tearing into our treat as we walked, she suggested the best way to enjoy food and also get the most out of it—sit down and savor.

It sounds simple. But think about how often you eat in front of the refrigerator, on the couch, or while walking around. One of the greatest signs we're overly hungry is when we eat whatever we can find, no matter where we are.

My clients talk a lot about the many places they eat. When I asked Jeff, one of my single clients, where he eats most often at home, he paused for a moment. "At work," he told me, "I eat at my desk. But at home, I lean against the counter and watch TV. I never sit down." And that often meant that he reached for another helping, just because it was right there next to him on the kitchen counter.

Time and again studies show that *where* you eat plays an important role in eating well and managing hunger. In one study, Canadian researchers divided people into two groups. One group ate food out of a plastic container standing up—like many of us. The other group ate a meal while sitting down at a table. When given their next meal a few hours later, the group that ate standing ate 30 percent more. Another study showed that parents of children who eat dinner at a kitchen table have lower body mass index (BMI).[125] There may be many reasons for this lower BMI, but part of the reason is the greater focus we give to eating when we eat at a table.

"Well," some of my clients say, "I'm sitting when I watch TV and eat." But there's no magic benefit to just sitting while we eat. In fact, when we sit in front of a TV, we're distracted. We don't enjoy our food as much, because we don't pay as much attention to it. And we're not paying attention to our own body's signals that tell us when we've had enough.

How does sitting down to eat help? And why is it so important to sit at a table? Sitting at the table helps us to focus, to be less distracted, and to be more mindful of our portions.

Hangry to Happy

Get off your feet. Whenever you eat, find a place. Instead of scarfing down a slice of pizza while you walk, find a park bench. Go to the lunchroom, or find a chair at a party. Remember, you'll be more satisfied and eat a more mindful portion if you take some time to focus on your food.

Find a table. Where do you eat most often? Is there a table involved? Or is there a table that *could* be involved? Figure out where there are tables in your environment at home and at work. Then make it a point to sit down to eat at one as often as you can. And even if you can't always find a table, you can put yourself in a "table mentality" by using one of the exercises here.

Make a table. When a table's not available, create one. Move papers off your desk to have a quiet spot for lunch, or sit down on the couch without the television on.

Center yourself. The real trick: don't just sit. Be fully present, mentally and physically, before you dig in. Wherever you eat, take a moment to center yourself. Put your feet flat against the floor and repeat the motto "Time to eat, off my feet, I'll be present in my seat." Use this to center your attention on your food and ground yourself to the spot.

HACK YOUR HABITS #39: **S**LOWLY CHEW: PACE, DON'T RACE

"I eat so quickly, like I am shoveling down my food as fast as possible. Sometimes I barely taste it. Once, I almost choked on a piece of meat. I coughed and coughed. It was my wake-up call that I need to slow down and chew my food more thoroughly."

When it comes to chewing...

a) I don't pay attention to chewing.
b) I chew a few times, enough to be able to swallow.
c) I chew sufficiently.
d) I chew for a long time, making sure the bite is broken down.

I recently ate lunch with my friend. She told me about a problem she was having with her boyfriend, who was giving her a lot of grief. And as she ate, she was chopping, not chewing. It was clear, without any words at all, that she was angry. It reminded me again that how we eat reflects how we feel. And how we feel affects how we eat.

Think for a moment about how you chew.

Many of my clients who have strong cravings tell me that chewing falls low on their priority list. When they see food, how they'll chew it is nowhere on their radar screen. Often, the tastier the food, the quicker they eat. The result is that they don't even really taste what they are eating. So they end up overeating and sometimes not even enjoying the food. "You can eat an entire plate of food," I tell them, "and not taste one bite."

And believe it or not, chewing has a lot to do with it.

Chewing is like breathing. We don't think much about the process of doing it until something makes it a challenge. If you are walking up a hill and suddenly your breathing becomes more difficult, you start to focus on it and try to control it. It's the same thing with a tough steak. Until you have to work at gnawing on the meat, your awareness and attention isn't drawn to chewing. Most of the time, we chew and breathe on autopilot.

Chewing is important to avoid choking, as in my client's story above. And chewing helps your body process food. But chewing can also impact hanger more than you may realize.

In a review of sixteen studies on chewing, researchers found that slow chewing decreases not just our hunger, but how much we eat.[126] Why? Chewing doesn't just break up food. The act of chewing sends signals to the gut that activate hormones that prepare the body to process food. To back this up, several studies have looked at what happens when you chew food but don't really eat[127] or when you chew gum.[128] What those researchers have found is that even without actually consuming food, the act of chewing plays a role in managing hunger and appetite by priming the body to fully enjoy it.[129, 130]

Hangry to Happy

Set your intention. Before you start eating, tell yourself, *I'm going to chew more consciously.* Setting an intention helps you to focus better on mindful eating. Chewing each bite approximately twenty-five times is optimal, according to a large review of studies on chewing.[131]

Notice others. The next time you're eating with your family or out for a bite with friends, notice how much they chew. Some people eat slowly, while others scarf down the whole plate in one bite. Others are somewhere in between.

Cut your food into smaller pieces. Fast eaters don't just eat quickly. They also tend to take gigantic bites. If you're taking huge bites and swallowing quickly, you're probably not chewing your food well. This means almost-whole pieces of food are ending up in your stomach. Then it's up to your poor stomach to do the work that should have started in your mouth. And that can lead to stomachaches, heartburn, poor digestion, nausea, and weight gain. If you have this tendency, you're not alone. And one way to break the habit is to cut your food into smaller, more manageable bites. It's just simple math—if we cut our food into smaller pieces, we have to eat more bites—which means we eat more slowly. So try smaller pieces, and see how it slows your eating.[132] Try out different sizes—cut it into quarter-, nickel-, and dime-sized pieces. The good news: studies also show that when we take smaller mouthfuls, we eat less—whether we're consuming chocolate or soup.[133]

Create a mindful pause. Between chewing each bite, take a mindful pause. Some examples of mindful pauses are taking a breath, a drink, switching utensils, or putting your fork down for a moment.

HACK YOUR HABITS #40: SURVEY YOUR OPTIONS

"I am typically so hungry, I barely slow down enough to appreciate what I am eating!"

When I eat...

a) I just dig in.
b) I pause for a moment to appreciate how it looks.
c) I sometimes won't eat it if it doesn't look tasty.
d) I make sure my plate looks pretty.

I'm most likely to look at my food when it's presented like a work of art: a perfectly plated restaurant meal or an elaborate wedding cake. Perfect rows of French pastries with strawberries perched on top always make me pause. It's so natural I don't even think about it.

But when it comes to everyday foods, sometimes we don't even glance down at the sandwich we're gobbling or the hamburger we're pulling out of the bag.

Since caveman times, looking at our food before eating has been a survival instinct. We look to make sure it appears good or safe, based on the color and smell.

We've all taken something out of the refrigerator and thought, "Hmm, better throw that out. Doesn't look like it's still safe to eat."

But looking at our food isn't just a matter of safety. Turns out, looking at our food also affects how much we eat—and how satisfied we feel.

You'd think that we feel hungry just because we need nutrients. But when scientists ran studies in which they simply put food directly into people via feeding tubes, they found that people still felt hungry—even though they had all the nutrients they needed.[134] The process of looking at your food, picking up your fork, and opening your mouth is important, too.

Visual cues help us know whether we've eaten enough or not. If we see a pile of mashed potatoes that we haven't made a dent in on our plate, we think, "I haven't eaten much." But if our plate is licked clean, we might say, "Wow, I ate all that!"

And the words we say to ourselves about how much we've eaten also affect our level of satisfaction. When we tell ourselves we've eaten well, we actually feel fuller.

My mother used to say "Look before you leap."

And now I say "Look before you leap — into lunch!"

Take a close look at your food before you take even one bite.

Hangry to Happy

Do a double take. Before you eat, take a moment to pause and scan your food. Notice the portion size and overall appearance. Does it look appetizing? Are the fruits and vegetables crisp and ripe? What is the portion size? A lot? A little?

Choose your words. If you tell yourself, "This looks really satisfying," your brain is more likely to register it as so. Start a meal or snack by saying these words to yourself.

Pace yourself. During the meal, check out the visual cues to see how much you have eaten. How many chicken bones are stacked up? How much of the casserole is gone?

Save everything! With snacks, it helps to leave a visual cue of what you have just eaten, so you remember. We are notorious for having a poor memory of what we eat. Leave the protein bar wrapper on your desk or the empty bowl of chips on the table. Seeing that you just ate something will help you to feel more satiated for longer simply because you remember you ate it!

HACK YOUR HABITS #41: SAVOR EACH BITE

"I enjoy food, but I don't really savor it. I discovered this when I watched my wife eat a single bite of chocolate and enjoy it completely. I was thinking about the next piece of chocolate before I even finished the one I had."

When it comes to tasting my food:

a) I gobble up food when I eat.

b) I don't really taste food unless it is very flavorful.

c) I try to taste each bite.

d) I pay a lot of attention to the different tastes and textures of everything I eat.

Every Christmas, I trick people into savoring food. I make a batch of my special chocolate crinkle cookies, which are heavenly, in my opinion. I give each person I know only one—yes, just one!—not a dozen. I wrap it beautifully. And then I watch what happens.

To date, no one has ever just said "thanks" and popped their single cookie into their mouth without a thought. Instead, people strategize for quite some time about how they are going to eat this cookie to maximize their enjoyment. Some people pick a special time when they can give it their full attention: "I'm going to eat this at three, after my meeting, when I can really sit down in the quiet and enjoy it." Other people plot how to make the most of the experience: "I'm going to warm it up and then sit down with a cup of coffee."

The goal in savoring food is to become more discerning about your eating habits. It reminds me of buying running shoes. I bought my first pair because I liked the color: green. That's it. It was my only criterion. But since then I've become incredibly discerning about running shoes—how they fit, the weight, the breathability, the bounce. Not all running shoes, I've learned, are the same. Different shoes function in different ways. And good shoes took my running to an entirely different level.

It's the same with food. Sometimes we eat it because we like how it looks. But when we become discerning, we think about the how the food tastes in our mouth. Do you like the texture? Does it taste good? Does it power you up? Our choices become more refined, specific, and proactive.

One of my clients likes tomatoes. She particularly savors them when they are in season. She spends a lot of time picking them, choosing ones that are a specific red and appear to be perfectly ripe. The entire process from start to finish enhances the taste and enjoyment for her.

Our fast-food culture teaches us the opposite of savoring. We often have the box of chicken nuggets open and one popped into our mouth before we pull out of the fast-food line.

But studies have shown that savoring food doesn't just mean we get more enjoyment from every bite. Savoring also promotes mindful eating—which in turn reduces hanger.[135]

Hangry to Happy

Turn on your senses. The most important thing you can do before you take a bite is to use all five of your senses. To do this, imagine that what you're about to eat is a completely new food to you. You've never seen it before. Imagine what you would do.

> *Smell.* Breathe in the scent of what you are about to eat.
> *Look.* Observe how the food looks and what's appetizing about it.
> *Listen.* What sounds do you hear when you interact with the food? Snaps? Sizzle? Crunch?
> *Touch.* How does the food feel in your mouth? On your fingers as you pick it up? Smooth? Crunchy?
> *Taste.* Is it spicy? Bland? Cooked just right?

Savor the first bite. Research shows that our pleasure doesn't grow with each bite. Instead, the first bite tastes the best because we become "habituated" or used to the taste as we eat. Then pleasure declines with each additional bite. So to enjoy your food more, savor those first bites—and don't try to take too many more, because they won't increase your pleasure.[136] Just commit to being very tuned in to the first bite.[137] Ask yourself if you love it, hate it, or it's just okay.

Set the food stage. Part of savoring food is setting up the entire experience to your liking. We develop muscle memory for particular ways of eating that enhance enjoyment. For example, maybe you like to drink coffee out of your favorite mug, sitting on a lounge chair on your back porch, early in the morning. You hold the mug in a certain way. Or you warm up a cookie to just the right temperature before you eat it. Before you eat, consider what you might do to set the stage to make it more enjoyable.

Practice savoring. Research indicates that using all your senses helps you savor food—but that takes practice.[138] So try some experiments by taking small bites of contrasting foods. This can help refine your palate and tune in to the nuances of flavor. For example, cut up four different types of cheese—cheddar, Gouda, blue cheese, and Muenster. Take a small bite of each and determine which one you like best. Or nibble on slices of four different varieties of apple (Golden Delicious, Red Delicious, Granny Smith, and Gala) and rank them according to sweetness and how much you like them. Perhaps arrange on a plate bites of four different types of chocolate, ranging in percent of cocoa (25 percent, 35 percent, 55 percent, 72 percent). Or put different pieces of fruit on a skewer. Take each one off slowly and savor it. This is a fun party activity or one to practice on your own to become an expert on your taste buds.

Use the shut-eye effect. When you take away one of your senses, you rely more on the others. And that means that your sense of taste may be sharpened. Participants in a recent study were either blindfolded or ate normally. Those who ate in the dark rated the food more enjoyable—and they ate less.[139] So before you take a bite, close your eyes for a split second and tune in.

HACK YOUR HABITS #42: **S**HIFT YOUR FOCUS

"I know I'm supposed to focus on my food. But I'm also trying to figure out everything else going on in my life. And I can't focus on everything at once. So, often, food doesn't get any of my attention—even when I'm eating it."

When I eat, typically...

a) I am driving, talking on the phone, or texting, and paying very little attention to my food.
b) I become easily distracted.
c) I stop what I am doing and focus on my food.
d) I pay attention to each bite.

When you eat, just eat.

It's not just a Zen proverb, it's something that I say all the time to my clients. And something I say to myself. And my kids.

Because focusing on eating when we eat is not easy.

"I don't have time!" my clients tell me. "I only have a few minutes for lunch."

"It seems like a waste of time," others say. "I could be doing something else, too."

One way or another, their objections are always about the use of time. And that's understandable.

Every day is hectic. You are pulled in dozens of directions at once. You have emails pouring into your inbox every moment. Your phone is blowing up. And you still have a ton of errands to run.

But our distracted lives have serious consequences.

One of my clients was recently in a car accident. When I asked what happened, she looked down at her lap sheepishly. "I always feared food would kill me," she said. "But I didn't think it would be literally. I was reaching for a chip in the bag next to me while I was driving, and I swerved."

Eating in the car doesn't always lead to car accidents. But distracted eating often leads to feeling regretfull or hangry. Eating while distracted is well known to lead to overeating, as underscored by a recent review of a whopping twenty-four studies in the *American Journal of Clinical Nutrition*.[140]

Bland food can also cause hanger. But there's hope in a recent article in the journal *Psychological Science,* which suggests a simple secret for making food taste better.[141] It's not a new spice or ingredient, like the salt I always add to chocolate cookies to enhance the flavor. It's a behavioral shift: not multitasking while you eat.

In the study, researchers asked participants to remember a seven-digit number or one-digit number. They did this while tasting something salty, sweet, or sour. Then they rated the intensity of the flavor. Participants who had to remember more numbers while eating (a more difficult task, or "cognitive load") rated the flavors as less intense. They also ate more sweet and salty foods.

The conclusion? Multitasking reduces the taste of food. Why? Because your brain has to process everything at once, and the different sensory experiences compete with one another. And it's likely that this doesn't apply just to taste. Whenever you juggle many things at once, your senses are pulled in many different directions. When we play a game on our phones while we're watching a movie, we don't enjoy either one as much.

A study published in the journal *Appetite* did a deep dive into what keeps us distracted from our food.[142] And it found there are two forms of distraction connected with food—things that distract us from hunger and things that distract us from eating.

Researchers randomized participants into groups and asked them to eat while doing a driving simulation, watching television, talking with a researcher, or sitting alone with no distraction. The drivers were distracted from their hunger by driving. But they were also distracted from eating by driving. So they ate a small amount, mindlessly. Participants watching television were distracted from their hunger by the show. But they weren't distracted from eating. So they mindlessly ate a large amount. Subjects who interacted with the researchers were distracted from eating, but still aware of their hunger. They ate little, probably because it's awkward to eat alone while a stranger watches. And the group who ate completely alone had the attention to give to both their hunger and their eating—in other words, mindful eating.

One question my clients often ask is about distraction while eating—for instance, with the TV on. Many of my clients say that they simply like it. That's fine. For some people, it's impractical, or simply no fun, not to have the TV on.

The goal isn't simply to turn off the TV or eat in complete silence. Can you watch TV and focus on your food? Yes! Your brain is capable of that. In fact, I often have the TV on simply as background noise, even though I couldn't tell you what is on.

What doesn't work is when you get completely engrossed in a TV show—so you get to the bottom of the bowl and don't know how you got there.

Hangry to Happy

Less time means more focus. It's not about adding more time to your meal. It's about giving your meal all of your focus. Even if you've only got a minute to snack, that's okay. Just give it your undivided attention.

Turn off distracting sounds. Manage the sounds in your life—beeps, TV, music, or anything that might take your attention away from the moment.

Invite your mind to dinner. So often, we are eating while our thoughts are somewhere else—anywhere besides the table. Before you eat, consciously invite your mind to join you. You can do this by picking a spot on the table to anchor your mind, such as a particular glass or bowl on the table. When your thoughts wander, simply bring your gaze back to that spot. Give yourself permission to put other worries and thoughts aside, and dedicate your full attention to what you are eating.

Check in. Ask yourself "How much focus am I giving my food, right now?" A lot? A little? What is one step you can take to increase your focus? Close your eyes? Let go of something that is bothering you for a moment? Look closely at what is in front of you?

HACK YOUR HABITS #43: **S**TOP RIGHT NOW!

"Out of nowhere, my mind will start to think about the cold mac and cheese in the fridge. I begin to think about how it would taste if I warmed it up for a minute in the microwave. The gooey goodness and buttery noodles would be so amazing. I think about each forkful of cheesiness. Suddenly, I can't get it out of my mind."

As soon as I think about a food I crave . . .

a) I have to have it!!
b) If the craving is strong and persistent, I go for it.
c) I can manage my craving, and I crave only a few things.
d) I work through my cravings, answering them mindfully.

It starts out like this. You are typing on your computer when seemingly out of nowhere, your mind says "Chocolate."

Hmm, you think.

Then your mind keeps talking. "Hey," it says. "Sharon left salted caramel chocolate brownies in the break room today. They're chewy, gooey, and amazing. So soft and rich."

Believe it or not, this thought process has a name: The Elaborated-Intrusion Theory of desire.[143] Basically, it says that food cravings happen in two stages. First, we have a spontaneous thought or craving: *I want chips!* It's intrusive, which means it just pops into your head without permission and with enough vigor that it stays and pushes out other thoughts. Phase two is when you begin to think about the yummy sensory qualities of whatever thought has just intruded on your mind: *chips are so crunchy and salty on my tongue.*[144]

Voila! Your mind begins to spin into a full-on food craving.

Cravings aren't easy to manage. A lot of my clients start out by trying to use the tug-of-war approach against them. Like my client Mike. "Yes," he'd tell himself. "I want to dive into the Tupperware container of chocolate-chip cookies my wife made. But no, I don't think that it is a good idea because I'd eat six right now."

The problem was, his thought process didn't stop there.

Because the craving kept coming back. "But, yes, I want them," he'd be thinking. "They're right there. But I shouldn't. I can't stop at just one."

What happens next is unpredictable. Sometimes the craving takes over, and sometimes it doesn't. But because the tug-of-war approach often fails, Mike and my other clients end up feeling that they have little control once a craving takes hold.

Luckily, there are other strategies for dealing with cravings.

The key is answering cravings consciously.

Elaborated-Intrusion theory tells us that we can't control whether we have a craving—whether that first idea pops into our mind or not. But studies show that we can influence the intensity of a craving.[145] You can ramp it up or cool it down with your thoughts. That is all in your hands—or mind.

In a study on cravings, 249 women completed an online questionnaire about their most recent food-craving experience. It's no surprise that a third of participants reported that when they have thoughts about craving food, they begin to imagine those foods.[146]

Then the women described all kinds of strategies they had tried to cope with their cravings. One in particular helped keep them from eating in response to a craving.

The most important detail, it turned out, was where the mind went after the first craving thought appeared in their head. Women who told themselves "It's just a thought" were significantly better able to work through their craving than ones who didn't talk to themselves objectively about the craving.

My client Mike described the power of thoughts in terms of wanting a new car. Every now and then, he told me, the thought that he wants one pops into his mind. He can go one of two ways with it. Either he puts a stop to it as soon as it pops into his mind, by saying "It's just a thought. I can't really afford one right now." Or, he said, he can start to fantasize about what kind of car and details like engine size and color. When he goes this route, his desire skyrockets and he sometimes even goes to car lots and looks at cars for hours.

Just because you have a thought doesn't mean you have to answer it. We think about, and want, a lot of things. But we don't just rush out and get them at the first thought. Most of the time, we take our time, decide whether we really need the thing and can afford it, and make a decision. And the same can be true for food.

Hangry to Happy

Watch your thoughts. When the very first thought of a craving pops into your head, tell yourself *"It's just a thought."* Remember that just because you have a thought doesn't mean you have to respond to it—or even keep thinking about it. A thought is NOT a command.

Turn off your inner TV. Once you have a craving, your best bet for controlling its intensity is to avoid letting it take root in your imagination. Imagining the smell, taste, and texture only ramps up the craving. Instead, take your thoughts in a different direction, toward something else. It may even be useful to choose something in advance to occupy your mind when you have a craving—something you like to think about that also absorbs your mind, like a favorite sports team, TV show, or hobby.

HACK YOUR HABITS #44: **S**LOW THE FORK DOWN!

"I eat way too fast. I blame my husband. He eats without even pausing to breathe. It's like we race through a meal."

When I eat . . .

a) I inhale my food.
b) I sometimes eat way too quickly, particularly if I'm really hungry.
c) I eat at a normal pace, not too fast or slow.
d) I eat slowly. Often I'm the last one done.

"I burned the back of my throat yesterday," my client Theresa told me, "and it still hurts. I was taking spicy, roasted potatoes out of the oven and immediately took one to test. I didn't even let it cool for a second. I put food that had been cooking at 400 degrees right into my mouth without even pausing."

She burned her mouth so severely that it stung for days. But it was a wake-up call. "I have to slow down when I eat," she said. "Not just because I am going to hurt myself, but because I don't enjoy food at all at this pace."

Many of my clients eat quickly due to habit or the environment they're in. It's not just chewing quickly, which we talked about in a previous tip; it's putting food into your mouth at a rapid pace. Consider whether you have a five-minute meal or a twenty-minute one. Often, my fast-eating clients will talk about growing up in a home where meals were quick or on the go. This sets the baseline for how fast they are likely to eat as adults. Think for a moment about your household growing up. Were meals at a leisurely pace? Or were they hurried, rushed, and on-the-go?

Theresa talked about growing up in a very tense home. Tempers could flare between her parents at any moment. Her job was to clear the table after dinner. She noticed that if she ate quickly, she could escape to her room as fast as possible. This set the stage for Theresa to eat at a breakneck speed, a habit she had to work hard to undo.

Quick-eating habits can also be personality-based. Some people are into details. They naturally approach situations and tasks slowly. Others are all about getting it done—even eating. They tend to get very irritated by things that slow them down—like people driving too slowly in the fast lane or a slow internet server.

But the biggest culprit in fast eating is not the clock—it's other people. We tend to eat at the same rate as those around us. And this was the case for Theresa. She said her husband ate faster than anyone else she knew. And she often found herself matching his pace bite for bite without even realizing it. Telling him to slow down never worked. Instead, she learned to focus on controlling her own pace, not his.

Theresa wasn't alone in being affected by how fast other people eat. In one study, participants were given either Chex Mix or M&M's while watching a movie. It turns out that even *what people eat in movies we're watching* can affect us. Viewers ate more food when they saw characters eating than they did after a character stopped eating.[147]

And one of the big downfalls of eating fast is that study after study has shown that eating fast is a recipe for mindless eating.[148] Anything we do too quickly, we don't tend to do well. When we rush our work, we forget details. When we hurry through tests, we get more wrong answers. And sometimes the consequences are more serious. When we drive too fast, we're more likely to get into accidents, and the accidents are more likely to be serious.

Slowing down our eating has proven benefits. And one of the biggest is that it helps us remember what we ate. That may sound like a surprising "benefit," but remembering what we eat helps us feel more satisfied for longer—and eat less mindlessly. In one study, participants were asked to eat a bowl of soup quickly or slowly. Participants who consumed the soup slowly reported a greater increase in fullness, both at the end of the meal and during the meal. And after three hours, participants who had eaten the soup slowly remembered eating a larger portion. These findings suggest that eating slowly promotes feeling more satisfied—and, more important, it helps us remember *feeling* satisfied. When we remember feeling satisfied, it's easier to eat more mindfully at the next meal, because meals and snacks that leave you satisfied leave a lasting mental imprint.[149]

Hangry to Happy

Set your intention. When you drive a car, you check the speed limit. So set your intended speed when you sit down to eat. Say to yourself "Pace, not race."

Choose your position. We often eat hunched over our plates, which shortens the distance between the fork and the plate. To slow down, place your back firmly against the back of your chair and sit up straight.

Pay attention to your partner. If you are eating with someone, take a moment to notice how quickly that person is eating. Fast? Moderate? Slow? Now, consciously determine whether you want to eat faster than, slower than, or at the same rate as your companion. It's polite to wait for everyone at the table to have food in front of them before digging in. Not only is this good manners, but it can also help people pace themselves so one member of a group isn't done long before the others, which tempts them to continue to eat until others are done, too. And remember, just because you all start at the same time doesn't mean you have to finish simultaneously.

X marks the spot. Need a moment to pause? Put your fork and knife down on your plate crossed over each other in the shape of an *X*. Focus your attention on that *X* for a moment to slow you down.

HACK YOUR HABITS #45: SMILE BETWEEN EACH BITE

"Mindful eating seriously changed my life. I went from a dieter who fretted and sweated about every calorie to someone who started to enjoy eating again. Every meal wasn't a judgment about myself as a person — I skipped the french fries so I am 'good' or I had two pieces of chocolate cake so I am 'bad.' Feeling good about how I eat makes me feel good about me. Period."

My general feeling about eating is that . . .

a) I find it very stressful.
b) I worry occasionally about what I eat.
c) I enjoy eating most of the time.
d) I love eating and it always makes me happy, without any stress.

I love the reaction I get when I reveal this last tip.
"Smile between bites," I tell my clients.

And they automatically smile in reaction to just receiving this happy advice. Sometimes they don't even really realize they do it.

I don't suggest this just because it creates a pause between bites to check in with yourself—which it does. Being happier when we eat has all kinds of other benefits as well.

In one recent study, researchers asked participants to eat either chocolate or crackers, either mindfully or without thinking much about it.[150] What they found did not surprise me. Participants who were instructed to eat mindfully had a greater increase in positive mood compared to participants who weren't— regardless of which food they picked. No matter what we eat, we can increase our happiness by eating it mindfully. Mindfully approaching anything we do increases our pleasure in it.

Smiling also kicks off an internal neurobiological response. When we smile, we actually feel happier—even if we weren't feeling happy to begin with. The facial feedback hypothesis offers a possible explanation for this: our brain recognizes the muscle movement as a smile and sends out happy chemicals to match. Try it right now! Smile widely to yourself. How do you feel?

Researchers have even studied how smiling might change cravings in healthy young women. They exposed sixty women to tasty food, then asked them to smile. The result: the women who smiled felt better able to handle their cravings.[151] It's research that might be particularly effective for people who are prone to emotional eating. But all of us can put it to work in our own lives, simply by smiling.

Hangry to Happy

Start with a smile. *"Peace begins with a smile."*—*Mother Teresa.*
I like this quote because it is true in your relationship with

food. Between bites, pause for a moment to smile. It can be any kind of smile. A closed-mouth Buddha-like smile or a big Cheshire Cat one. Whatever works for you.

Take a moment. Take a bite. Smile. Smiling gives you a moment to pause. In that pause time space, think. Do you want the next bite? Or are you satisfied by this one? Then, decide. Repeat.

SUMMARY OF HACK YOUR HABITS

In this chapter, you learned about what I call the "hows" of mindful eating. They're focused less on *what* you are eating and more on the *way you eat*. Even the seemingly smallest actions, like picking up your fork, choosing a place to sit, pausing before a bite, or eating slowly, have a big impact on the experience of eating.

My hope is that you acquire a new mindfulness of the entire eating pathway, start to finish — from the moment the idea to eat pops into your head to putting down your napkin and pushing away your plate. And I hope that mindfulness will give you new happiness whenever you eat.

Here's a checklist of the 10 *S*'s of mindful eating we just discussed. Put a check mark by the things you do well and an *X* by actions that may need more of your mindful attention.

Whether you are just beginning mindful eating or an expert, these all take practice. Stick with it!

___ Do I mindfully/consciously select food?
___ Do I try new things when I eat?
___ Do I sit down when I eat?
___ Do I chew a sufficient number of times?

__ Do I consciously think through all my food options?

__ Do I savor each bite?

__ Do I give eating my full attention?

__ Do I stop eating when I am satisfied?

__ Do I eat at a slow rate?

__ Do I take a happy pause between each bite?

Congratulations!

You made it to the very end of this book—hopefully without getting hangry. (If you did get hungry, that's okay!) At this juncture, you know exactly what to do to turn that hanger into happiness.

My hope is that you are actually content and happy right now, in this very moment. Not just your stomach, but your mind. I feel excited and motivated whenever I learn new things, and I bet you do, too.

It's likely that you've already had some aha! moments that have led you to try mindful eating. If not, it's time to start putting what you've learned into practice.

I would love to hear from you. Seriously. You can find my contact information on my website. People write to me all the time, from all over the world. They share what they were thinking and doing *before* the Hanger Management program and how Hanger Management tools and skills have changed their life for the better!

Alas, only so much can fit into a book. To learn more about my psychology practice and the other eight books I've written, and to grab your free resources and downloads, I welcome you to please visit my website, eatingmindfully.com, anytime!

I wish you well, and as always, a mindful journey forward.
Let go of hanger.
Eat, drink, and be mindful!

Mindfully yours,
Dr. Susan Albers

Acknowledgments

Thank you!

I'd like to extend a mindful thank you to the following people...

My awesome family—Brooke, Jack, and John. My parents, Thomas and Carmela, and sisters, Linda and Angie. As well as John, Rhonda, Jim, and Ashley.

Dr. Joe Tatta and Dr. Nicole Beurkens, who are not only my colleagues—they have become incredible collaborators, brainstorm buddies, and my very good friends.

Jaidree Braddix and Celeste Fine at Park & Fine Literary and Media for helping turn my ideas into actual books on the shelves.

A humble thank-you to the fans of mindful eating—readers, clients, and social media followers. As always, I am honored to be a part of your life.

A special thank-you to the professionals who tirelessly work to help people transform their relationships with food every day. You improve the quality of people's lives exponentially and help them to truly enjoy food—as they should!

A grateful thank-you to Kelly Taylor for helping people find my books and take notice of them!

An appreciative thank-you to Marisa Vigilante and the team at Little, Brown Spark, Hachette Book Group, for taking on this book and introducing Hanger Management to the world.

My gratitude to Chelsea Denlinger for her amazing social

media ideas, Alejandra Ortega for technical support, Randy Berry for inspiring creative writing, F.H. for encouraging motivation, and Carey Wallace for editing assistance.

And finally, those who add fun, adventure, and a supportive ear: Victoria Gould, Susan Heady, Betsy Swope, Jane Lindquist Lesniewski, and the Lingenfelter, Wright, Burgett, Barr, and Grassman families.

Notes

1. B. J. Bushman et al., "Low glucose relates to greater aggression in married couples," *Proceedings of the National Academy of Sciences of the United States of America* 111, no.17 (April 14, 2014): 6254–6274. doi.org/10.1073/pnas.1400619111.

2. Shai Danziger, Jonathan Levav, and Liora Avnaim-Pesso, "Extraneous factors in judicial decisions," *Proceedings of the National Academy of Sciences of the United States of America* 108, no. 17 (April 26, 2011): 6889–6892. doi.org/10.1073/pnas.1018033108.

3. Andreas Glöckner, "The irrational hungry judge effect revisited: Simulations reveal that the magnitude of the effect is overestimated," *Judgment and Decision Making* 11, no. 6 (November 2016): 601–610. http://journal.sjdm.org/16/16823/jdm16823.pdf.

4. Rozita H Anderberg et al., "The Stomach-Derived Hormone Ghrelin Increases Impulsive Behavior," *Neuropsychopharmacology* 141 (October 1, 2015): 1199–1209. doi.org/10.1038/npp.2015.297.

5. Alexa Hoyland, Louise Dye, and Clare L. Lawton, "A systematic review of the effect of breakfast on the cognitive performance of children and adolescents," *Nutrition Research Reviews* 22, no. 2 (December 2009): 220–243. doi.org/10.1017/S0954422409990175.

6. Katie Adolphus, Clare L. Lawton, Claire L. Champ, and Louise Dye, "The Effects of Breakfast and Breakfast Composition on Cognition in Children and Adolescents: A Systematic Review," *Nutrition* 7, no. 3 (May 2016): 590S–612S. doi.org/10.3945/an.115.010256.

7. Pippa Wysong, "Breakfast Enhances Cognition in Children and Adolescents," *BOLD: Blog on Learning and Development,* September 29, 2017.

8. Takaaki Komiyama et al., "Cognitive function at rest and during exercise following breakfast omission," *Physiology and Behavior* 157 (April 1, 2016): 178–184. doi.org/10.1016/j.physbeh.2016.02.013.

9. Neil Bernard Boyle, Clare Louise Lawton, and Louise Dye, "The Effects of Carbohydrates, in Isolation and Combined with Caffeine, on Cognitive Performance and Mood—Current Evidence and Future Directions," *Nutrients* 10, no. 2 (February 2018): 192. doi.org/10.3390/nu10020192.

10. Michael Macht and Dorothee Dettmer, "Everyday mood and emotions after eating a chocolate bar or an apple," *Appetite* 46, no. 3 (May 2006): 332–336. doi.org/10.1016/j.appet.2006.01.014.

11. E. F. Coccaro, R. Lee, T. Liu, and A. A. Mathé, "Cerebrospinal fluid neuropeptide Y-like immunoreactivity correlates with impulsive aggression in human subjects," *Biological Psychiatry* 72, no. 12 (December 15, 2012): 997–1003. doi.org/10.1016/j.biopsych.2012.07.029.

12. Silvia U Maier et al., "Acute Stress Impairs Self-Control in Goal-Directed Choice," *Cell.com* 87, no. 3 (August 5, 2015): 621–631. doi.org/10.1016/j .neuron.2015.07.005.

13. Jennifer K. MacCormack and Kristen A. Lindquist, "Feeling hangry? When hunger is conceptualized as emotion," *Emotion* 19, no. 2 (March 2019): 301–319. doi.org/10.1037/emo0000422.

14. Honor Whiteman, "Sleep deprivation increases hunger in similar way to marijuana," *Medical News Today* (March 1, 2016). https://www.medical newstoday.com/articles/307203.php?utm_source=Medical News Today.

15. Marie-Pierre St.-Onge, Anja Mikic, and Cara E. Pietrolungo, "Effects of Diet on Sleep Quality," *Advances in Nutrition* 7, no. 5 (September 15, 2016): 938–949. doi.org/10.3945/an.116.012336.

16. Jean-Philippe Chaput and Angelo Tremblay, "Adequate sleep to improve the treatment of obesity," *Canadian Medical Association Journal* 184, no. 18 (December 2012): 1975–1976. doi.org/10.1503/cmaj.120876.

17. Haya K. Al Khatib et al., "Sleep extension is a feasible lifestyle intervention in free-living adults who are habitually short sleepers: a potential strategy for decreasing intake of free sugars? A randomized controlled pilot study," *American Journal of Clinical Nutrition* 17, no. 1 (January 2018): 43–53. doi.org/10.1093/ajcn/nqx030.

18. Damien Leger, Virginie Bayon, and Alice de Sanctis, "The role of sleep in the regulation of body weight," *Molecular and Cellular Endocrinology* 418, pt. 2 (December 15, 2015): 101–107. doi.org/10.1016/j.mce.2015.06.030.

19. Filip Ottosson et al., "Connection Between BMI-Related Plasma Metabolite Profile and Gut Microbiota," *The Journal of Clinical Endocrinology & Metabolism* 103, no. 4 (February 1, 2018): 1491–1501. doi.org/10.1210 /jc.2017-02114.

20. Caroline J. K. Wallace and Roumen Milev, "The effects of probiotics on depressive symptoms in humans: a systematic review," *Annals of General Psychiatry* 16 (February 20, 2017). doi.org/10.1186/s12991-017-0138-2.

21. Carolyn Gregoire, "Sauerkraut Could Be the Secret to Curing Social Anxiety," *Huffington Post Science,* June 10, 2015. https://www.huffington post.com/2015/06/10/probiotics-gut-bacteria-a_n_7545942.html.

22. K. Tillisch et al., "Consumption of fermented milk product with probiotic modulates brain activity," *Gastroenterology* 144, no. 7 (June 2013): 1394–1401. doi.org/10.1053/j.gastro.2013.02.043.

23. Ioana A. Marin et al., "Microbiota alteration is associated with the development of stress-induced despair behavior," *Scientific Reports* 7, article no. 43859 (2017). doi.org/10.1038/srep43859.

24. Erin Frey and Todd Rogers, "Persistence: How Treatment Effects Persist After Interventions Stop," *Policy Insights from the Behavioral and Brain Sciences* 1, no. 1 (2014): 172–179. doi.org/10.1177/2372732214550405.

25. Samuel L. Buckner, Paul D. Loprinzi, and Jeremy P. Loenneke, "Why don't more people eat breakfast? A biological perspective," *The American Journal of Clinical Nutrition* 103, no. 6 (June 2016): 1555–1556. doi.org/10.3945/ajcn.116.132837.

26. E. M. Ackuaku-Dogbe and B. Abaidoo, "Breakfast eating habits among medical students," *Ghana Medical Journal* 48, no. 2 (2014): 66–70.

27. A. P. Goldstone et al., "Fasting biases brain reward systems towards high-calorie foods," *European Journal of Neuroscience* 30, no. 8 (October 2009): 1625–1635. doi.org/10.1111/j.1460-9568.2009.06949.x.

28. A. Lesani, A. Mohammadpoorasi, J. M. Esfeh, and A. Fakhari, "Eating breakfast, fruit and vegetable intake and their relation with happiness in college students," *Eating and Weight Disorders* 21, no. 4 (December 2016): 645–651. https://www.ncbi.nlm.nih.gov/pubmed/26928281.

29. Jerica M. Berge et al., "Intergenerational Transmission of Parent Encouragement to Diet from Adolescence into Adulthood," *Pediatrics* 141, no. 4 (April 2018). doi.org/10.1111/10.1542/peds.2017-2955.

30. Anika Küppel, Martin J. Shipley, Clare H. Llewellyn, and Eric J. Brunner, "Sugar intake from sweet food and beverages, common mental disorder and depression: prospective findings from the Whitehall II study," *Scientific Reports* 7, no. 1 (July 27, 2017). doi.org/10.1038/s41598-017-05649-7.

31. Larissa Ledochowski, Gerhard Ruedl, Adrian H. Taylor, and Martin Kopp, "Acute Effects of Brisk Walking on Sugary Snack Cravings in Overweight People, Affect and Responses to a Manipulated Stress Situation and to a Sugary Snack Cue: A Crossover Study," *PLOS One* 10, no. 3 (March 11, 2015). doi.org/10.1371/journal.pone.0119278.

32. James E. Gangwisch et al., "High glycemic index diet as a risk factor for depression: analyses from the Women's Health Initiative," *The American Journal of Clinical Nutrition* 102, no.2 (August 2015): 454–463. doi.org/10.3945/ajcn.114.103846.

33. Beatrice A. Golomb, Marcella A. Evans, Halbert L. White, and Joel E. Dimsdale, "Trans Fat Consumption and Aggression," *PLOS One* 7, no. 3 (2012). doi.org/10.1371/journal.pone.0032175.

34. J. E. Flood-Obbagy and B. J. Rolls, "The effect of fruit in different forms on energy intake and satiety at a meal," *Appetite* 52, no. 2 (April 2009): 416–422. doi.org/10.1016/j.appet.2008.12.001.

35. Caroline J. Edmonds, Rosanna Crombie, Haiko Ballieux, Mark R. Gardner, Lynne Dawkins, "Water consumption, not expectancies about water

consumption, affects cognitive performance in adults," *Appetite* 60 (November 16, 2013): 148–153. doi.org/10.1016/j.appet.2016.11.011.

36. C. X. Muñoz et al., "Habitual total water intake and dimensions of mood in healthy young women." *Appetite* 92 (September 2015): 81–86. doi .org/10.1016/j.appet.2015.05.002.

37. Charles Spence, Betina Piqueras-Fiszman, Charles Michel, and Ophelia Deroy, "Plating manifesto (II): the art and science of plating," *Flavour* 3, no. 4 (2014). doi.org/10.1186/2044-7248-3-4.

38. Jessica Rowley and Charles Spence, "Does the visual composition of a dish influence the perception of portion size and hedonic preference?," *Appetite* 128 (September 1, 2018): 79–86. doi.org/10.1016/j.appet.2018.06.005.

39. Vanessa Harrar, Betina Piqueras-Fiszman, and Charles Spence, "There's more to taste in a coloured bowl," *Perception* 40, no. 7 (January 1, 2011): 880–882. doi.org/10.1068/p7040.

40. Arianna McClain et al., "Visual illusions and plate design: the effects of plate rim widths and rim coloring on perceived food portion size," *International Journal of Obesity* 38, no. 5 (May 2014): 657–662. doi.org/10.1038 /ijo.2013.169.

41. Jennifer A. Hunter, Gareth J. Hollands, Dominique-Laurent Couturier, and Theresa M. Marteau, "Effect of snack-food proximity on intake in general population samples with higher and lower cognitive resource," *Appetite* 121 (February 2018): 337–347. doi.org/10.1016/j.appet.2017.11.101.

42. Billy Langlet et al., "Objective quantification of the food proximity effect on grapes, chocolate and cracker consumption in a Swedish high school. A temporal analysis," *PLOS One* (August 10, 2017). doi.org/10.1371/jour nal.pone.0182172.

43. Paul Rozin et al., "Nudge to Nobesity I: Minor changes in accessibility decrease food intake, *Judgment and Decision Making* 6, no. 4 (June 2011): 323–332. http://journal.sjdm.org/11/11213/jdm11213.html.

44. Dianne Engell et al., "Effects of effort and social modeling on drinking in humans," *Appetite* 26, no. 2 (April 1996): 129–138. doi.org/10.1006 /appe.1996.0011.

45. Rosemary Walmsley et al., "Choice architecture modifies fruit and vegetable purchasing in a university campus grocery store: time series modelling of a natural experiment," *BMC Public Health* 18 (2018). doi .org/10.1186/s12889-018-6063-8.

46. Susmita Baral, "How Binge Watching Affects Our Eating Habits," *NPR: The Salt* (December 31, 2015). https://www.npr.org/sections/thesalt /2015/12/31/461594989/netflix-and-chew-how-binge-watching-affects- our-eating-habits.

47. Ryan Dwyer, Kostadin Kushlev, and Elizabeth Dunn, "Smartphone use undermines enjoyment of face-to-face social interactions," *Journal of*

Experimental Social Psychology 78 (November 2017). doi.org/10.1016/j .jesp.2017.10.007.

48. Melanie Dadourian, "One third of Americans can't eat without their cell phones, study finds," *Fox News* (January 23, 2018). https://www.foxnews .com/health/one-third-of-americans-cant-eat-without-their -cellphones-study-finds.

49. Adrian F. Ward, Kristen Duke, Ayelet Gneezy, and Maarten W. Bos, "Brain Drain: the mere presence of one's own smartphone reduces available cognitive capacity," *Journal of the Association for Consumer Research* 2, no. 2 (April 2017). doi.org/10.1086/691462.

50. Cary Stothart, Ainsley Mitchum, and Courtney Yehnert, "The attentional cost of receiving a cell phone notification," *Journal of Experimental Psychology: Human Perception and Performance* 41, no. 4 (August 2015): 893–897. dx.doi.org/10.1037/xhp0000100.

51. Jane Ogden et al., "'Snack' versus 'meal': The impact of label and place on food intake," *Appetite* 120 (January 1, 2018): 666–672. doi.org/10.1016/j .appet.2017.10.026.

52. Sungeun Cho et al., "Blue lighting decreases the amount of food consumed in men, but not in women," *Appetite* 85 (February 1, 2015): 111–117. doi.org/10.1016/j.appet.2014.11.020.

53. Aimee Hassenbeck et al., "Color and illuminance of lighting can modulate willingness to eat bell peppers," *Journal of the Science of Food and Agriculture* (December 6, 2013). doi.org/10.1002/jsfa.6523.

54. Erhard Lick, Bettina König, Monyédodo Régis Kpossa, and Violetta Buller, "Sensory expectations generated by colours of red wine labels," *Journal of Retailing and Consumer Services* 37 (July 2017): 146–158. doi .org/10.1016/j.jretconser.2016.07.005.

55. Leonie Reutner, Oliver Genschow, and Michaela Wänke, "The adaptive eater: perceived healthiness moderates the effect of the color red on consumption," *Food Quality and Preference* 44 (September 2015): 172–178. doi .org/10.1016/j.foodqual.2015.04.016.

56. Meng Shen, Lijia Shi and Zhifeng Gao, "How does color affect attention to information on food labels and preference for food attributes?," *Food Quality and Preference* 64 (March 2018): 47–55. doi.org/10.1016/j .foodqual.2017.10.004.

57. Milica Vasilijevic, Rachel Pechey, and Theresa M. Marteau, "Making food labels social: The impact of colour of nutritional labels and injunctive norms on perceptions and choice of snack foods," *Appetite* 91 (August 2016): 56–63. doi.org/10.1016/j.appet.2015.03.034.

58. Oliver Genschow, Leonie Reutner, and Michaela Wänke, "The color red reduces snack food and soft drink intake," *Appetite* 58, no. 2 (April 2012): 669–702. doi.org/10.1016/j.appet.2011.12.023.

59. Jonathan P. Schuldt, "Does green mean healthy? Nutrition label color affects perceptions of healthfulness," *Health Communication* 28, no. 8 (February 27, 2013): 814–821. doi.org/10.1080/10410236.2012.725270.

60. A. N. Thorndike, J. Riis, L. M. Sonnenberg, and D. E. Levy, "Traffic-light labels and choice architecture: promoting healthy food choices," *American Journal of Preventative Medicine* 46, no. 2 (February 2014): 143–149. doi.org/10.1016/j.amepre.2013.10.002.

61. Robert M. Siegel et al., "Emoticon Use Increases Plain Milk and Vegetable Purchase in a School Cafeteria without Adversely Affecting Total Milk Purchase," *Clinical Therapy* 37, no. 9 (September 1, 2015): 1938–1943. doi.org/10.1016/j.clinthera.2015.07.016.

62. C. A. Richards and A. G. Rundle, "Business Travel and Self-rated Health, Obesity, and Cardiovascular Disease Risk Factors," *Journal of Occupational and Environmental Medicine* 53, no. 4 (April 2011): 358–363. doi.org/10.1097/JOM.0b013e3182143e77.

63. Milenko Martinovich, "Decadent-sounding descriptions could lead to higher consumption of vegetables, Stanford research finds," *Stanford News* (June 21, 2017). https://news.stanford.edu/press-releases/2017/06/12/decadent-sounding-labeling-may-lead-people-eat-vegetables/.

64. Vanessa Alom et al., "Breaking bad habits by improving executive function in individuals with obesity," *BMC Public Health* 18 (April 16, 2018): 505. doi.org/10.1186/s12889-018-5392-y.

65. Susan Churchill, Donna C. Jessop, Ricky Green, and Peter R. Harris, "Self-affirmation improves self-control over snacking among participants low in eating self-efficacy," *Appetite* 123 (April 1, 2018): 264–268. doi.org/10.1016/j.appet.2017.12.028.

66. Elena Holmes, "McDonald's tap tech to drive World Cup orders," *Sports Pro Media* (July 2, 2018). http://www.sportspromedia.com/news/mcdonalds-tech-world-cup-hungry-moments.

67. "McDonald's Partners with Google to Anticipate 'Hungry Moments'," *Sports Business Daily Global* Issues (July 3, 2018). https://www.sportsbusinessdaily.com/Global/Issues/2018/07/03/World-Cup/McDonalds.aspx.

68. John M. Kearny and Sinead McElhone, "Perceived barriers in trying to eat healthier—results of a pan-EU consumer attitudinal survey," *British Journal of Nutrition* 81, no. 2 (May 1999): S133–137. doi.org/10.1017/S0007114599000987.

69. Laura C. Ortinau, Heather A. Hoertel, Steve M. Douglas, and Heather J. Leidy, "Effects of high-protein vs. high-fat snacks on appetite control, satiety, and eating initiation in healthy women," *Nutrition Journal* 13 (2014). doi.org/10.1186/1475-2891-13-97.

70. Adrian Meule and Andrea Kebler, "A Pilot Study on the Effects of Slow Paced Breathing on Current Food Craving," *Applied Psychophysiology and Biofeedback* 42, no.1 (2017): 59–68. doi.org/10.1007/s10484-017-9351-7.

71. Rebecca G. Boswell, Wendy Sun, Shosuke Suzuki, and Hedy Kober, "Training in cognitive strategies reduces eating and improves food choice," *Proceedings of the National Academy of Sciences of the United States of America* 115, no. 48 (November 12, 2018): E11238–E11247. doi.org /10.1073/pnas.1717092115.

72. J. K. Kiecolt-Glaser et al., "Depressive symptoms, omega-6:omega-3 fatty acids, and inflammation in older adults," *Psychosomatic Medicine* 69, no. 3 (April 2007): 217–224. doi.org/10.1097/PSY.0b013e3180313a45.

73. "Deep forehead wrinkles may signal a higher risk for cardiovascular mortality," *ScienceDaily* (August 26, 2018). https://www.sciencedaily.com /releases/2018/08/180826120738.htm.

74. Noura S. Dosoky and William N. Setzer, "Biological activities and safety of *Citrus* spp. Essential Oils," *International Journal of Molecular Sciences* 19, no. 7 (1966). doi.org/10.3390/ijms19071966.

75. A. Steptoe et al., "The Effects of Tea on Physiological Stress Responsivity and Post-Stress Recovery: A Randomised Double-Blind Trial," *Psychopharmacology* 190, no. 1 (January 2007): 81–89. https://www.ncbi.nlm.nih .gov/pubmed/17013636.

76. Kris Gunnars, "Proven Health Benefits of Dark Chocolate," *Healthline* (June 25, 2018). https://www.healthline.com/nutrition/7-health-benefits -dark-chocolate.

77. B. O. Rennard et al., "Chicken soup inhibits neutrophil chemotaxis in vitro," *Chest* 118, no. 4 (October 2000): 1150–1157. doi.org/10.1378/chest.118.4.1150.

78. Katie Adolphus, Clare L. Lawton, Claire Champ, and Louise Dye, "The Effects of Breakfast and Breakfast Composition on Cognition in Children and Adolescents: A Systematic Review," *Advances in Nutrition* 7, no.3 (May 2016): 590S–612S. doi.org/10.3945/an.115.010256.

79. Eiichi Yoshimura, Yoichi Hatamoto, Satomi Yonekura, and Hiroaki Tanaka, "Skipping breakfast reduces energy intake and physical activity in healthy women who are habitual breakfast eaters: A randomized crossover trial," *Physiology and Behavior* 174 (May 15, 2017): 89–94. doi.org/10.1016/j .physbeh.2017.03.008.

80. Derrick Brown and Matthew Wyon, "The effect of moderate glycemic energy bar consumption on blood glucose and mood in dancers," *Medical problems of performing artists* 29, no. 1 (March 2014): 27–31. doi.org/10 .21091/mppa.2014.1007.

81. Mary Brophy Marcus, "Could a healthier diet help you sleep better?," CBSNews.com (February 10, 2016): https://www.cbsnews.com/news /could-a-healthier-diet-improve-sleep/.

82. Marie-Pierre St.-Onge, Amy Roberts, Ari Schecter, and Arindam Roy Choudhury, "Fiber and Saturated Fat Are Associated with Sleep Arousals and Slow Wave Sleep," *Journal of Clinical Sleep Medicine* 15, no. 5 (January 2016): 19–24. doi.org/10.5664/jcsm.5384.

83. Marsha McCulloch, "The 15 Best Healthy Late-Night Snacks," *Healthline* (June 24, 2018). https://www.healthline.com/nutrition/healthy-late-ni ght-snacks.

84. Marie-Pierre St.-Onge, Anja Mikic, and Cara E. Pietrolungo, "Effects of Diet on Sleep Quality," *Advances in Nutrition* 7, no. 5 (September 2016): 938–949. doi.org/10.3945/an.116.012336.

85. Juliet M. Pullar, Anitra C. Carr, Stephanie M. Bozonet, and Margreet C. M. Vissers, "High Vitamin C Status Is Associated with Elevated Mood in Male Tertiary Students," *Antioxidants (Basel)* 7, no. 7 (July 2018): 91. doi .org/10.3390/antiox7070091.

86. Kate L. Brookie, Georgia I. Best, and Tamlin S. Conner, "Intake of Raw Fruits and Vegetables Is Associated with Better Mental Health Than Intake of Processed Fruit and Vegetables," *Frontiers in Psychology* (April 10, 2018). doi.org/10.3389/fpsyg.2018.00487.

87. Alice G. Walton, "Dark Chocolate May Boost Brain Function, Immunity and Mood," *Forbes* (April 27, 2018). https://www.forbes.com/sites/aliceg walton/2018/04/27/dark-chocolate-may-boost-brain-function-immunity -and-mood/#2e3e6da04608.

88. Robert Krikorian et al., "Blueberry Supplementation Improves Memory in Older Adults," *Journal of Agricultural and Food Chemistry* 58, no. 7 (January 4, 2010). doi.org/10.1021/jf9029332.

89. Katie L. Barfoot et al., "The effects of acute wild blueberry supplementation on the cognition of 7–10-year-old schoolchildren," *European Journal of Nutrition* (October 16, 2018): 1–10. doi.org/10.1007/s00394-018-1843-6.

90. Farzaneh A. Sorond et al., "Neurovascular coupling, cerebral white matter integrity, and response to cocoa in older people," *Neurology* 81, no. 10 (September 3, 2013). doi.org/10.1212/WNL.0b013e3182a351aa.

91. Lee Berk et al., **"Dark chocolate (70% organic cacao) increases acute and chronic EEG power spectral density (μV^2) response of gamma frequency (25–40 Hz) for brain health: enhancement of neuroplasticity, neural synchrony, cognitive processing, learning, memory, recall, and mindfulness meditation," *The FASEB Journal* (April 20, 2018). https://www.fasebj .org/doi/10.1096/fasebj.2018.32.1_supplement.878.10.

92. Selvaraju Subash et al., "Neuroprotective effects of berry fruits on neuro-degenerative diseases," *Neural Regeneration Research* 9, no. 16 (August 15, 2014): 1557–1566. doi.org/10.4103/1673-5374.139483.

93. Raúl Domínguez et al., "Effects of Beetroot Juice Supplementation on Cardiorespiratory Endurance in Athletes. A Systematic Review," *Nutrients* 9, no. 1 (January 2017). doi.org/10.3390/nu9010043.

94. E. L. Wightman et al., "Dietary nitrate modulates cerebral blood flow parameters and cognitive performance in humans: A double-blind, placebo-controlled, crossover investigation," *Physiology and Behavior* (October 1, 2015): 149–158. doi.org/10.1016/j.physbeh.2015.05.035.

95. Tennille D. Presley et al., "Acute effect of a high nitrate diet on brain perfusion in older adults," *Nitric Oxide* 24, no. 1 (January 1, 2011): 34–42. doi.org/10.1016/j.niox.2010.10.002.

96. Ludovico Alisi et al., "Between Vitamin K and Cognition: A Review of Current Evidence," *Frontiers in Neurology* (March 19, 2019): doi.org/10.3389/fneur.2019.00239.

97. Anders Schmidt et al., "Green tea extract enhances parieto-frontal connectivity during working memory processing," *Psychopharmacology* 231, no. 19 (2014): 3879–3888. doi.org/10.1007/s00213-014-3526-1.

98. David Christopher Nieman et al., "Bananas as an energy source during Exercise: A Metabolomics Approach," *PLOS One* 7, no. 5 (May 2012). doi.org/10.1371/journal.pone.0037479.

99. Channa Marsh, Daniel Green, Louise Taylor, and Kym J. Guelfi, "Consumption of dark chocolate attenuates subsequent food intake compared with milk and white chocolate in postmenopausal women," *Appetite* 116 (September 1, 2017): 544–551. doi.org/10.1016/j.appet.2017.05.050.

100. Sarah O. Hull et al., "A mid-morning snack of almonds generates satiety and appropriate adjustments of subsequent food intake in healthy women," *European Journal of Nutrition* 54, no. 5 (August 2015): 803–810. doi.org/10.1007/s00394-014-0759-z.

101. Steve Douglas, Laura C. Ortinau, Heather A. Hoertel, and Heather Leidy, "Low, moderate, or high protein yogurt snacks on appetite control and subsequent eating in healthy women," *Appetite* 60, no. 1 (September 2012): 117–122. doi.org/10.1016/j.appet.2012.09.012.

102. Heather J. Leidy, Laura C. Ortinau, Steve M. Douglas, and Heather A. Hoertel, "Beneficial effects of a higher-protein breakfast on the appetitive, hormonal, and neural signals controlling energy intake regulation in overweight/obese, 'breakfast-skipping,' late-adolescent girls," *American Journal of Clinical Nutrition* 97, no. 4 (April 2013): 677–688. doi.org/10.3945/ajcn.112.053116.

103. Jillon S. Vander Wal et al., "Short-Term Effect of Eggs on Satiety in Overweight and Obese Subjects," *Journal of the American College of Nutrition* 24, no. 6 (December 2005): 510–515.

104. Helen M. Parretti et al., "Efficacy of water preloading before main meals as a strategy for weight loss in primary care patients with obesity," *Obesity* 23, no. 9 (September 2015): 1785–1791. doi.org/10.1002/oby.21167.

105. Robert A. Corney, Caroline Sunderland, and Lewis J. James, "Immediate pre-meal water ingestion decreases voluntary food intake in lean young males," *European Journal of Nutrition* 55, no. 2 (March 2016): 815–819. doi.org/10.1007/s00394-015-0903-4.

106. Catharine Paddock, "Two cups of water before each meal enhanced weight loss in clinical trials," *Medical News Today* (August 24, 2010). https://www.medicalnewstoday.com/articles/198720.php.

107. Ji Na Jeong, "Effect of Pre-meal Water Consumption on Energy Intake and Satiety in Non-obese Young Adults," *Clinical Nutrition Research* 7, no. 4 (October 2018): 291–296. doi.org/10.7762/cnr.2018.7.4.291.

108. Jordan Lite, "Vitamin D deficiency soars in the U.S., study says," *Scientific American* (March 23, 2009). https://www.scientificamerican.com/article/vitamin-d-deficiency-united-states/?redirect=1.

109. Ibrar Anjum et al., "The role of vitamin D in brain health: a mini literature review," *Cureus* 10, no. 7 (July 2018): e2960. doi.org/10.7759/cureus.2960.

110. Gleicilaine A. S. Casseb, Manuella P. Kaster, and Ana Lúcia S. Rodrigues, "Potential role of Vitamin D for the Management of Depression and Anxiety," *CNS Drugs* (May 15, 2019): 1–19. doi.org/10.1007/s40263-019-00640-4.

111. G. Bjorn et al., "Linking Vitamin D status, executive functioning, and self-perceived mental health in adolescents through multivariate analysis: a randomized double-blind placebo control trial," *Scandinavian Journal of Psychology* 58, no. 2 (April 2017): 123–130. doi.org/10.1111/sjop.12353.

112. "Vitamin D Supplements May Aid Weight Loss for Obese and Over-weight People, Study Finds," *Huffington Post UK* (August 5, 2015). https://www.huffingtonpost.co.uk/2015/05/08/vitamin-d-supplements-weight-loss-study_n_7239722.html?guccounter=2.

113. B. S. Peters et al., "The influence of breakfast and dairy products on dietary calcium and vitamin D intake in postpubertal adolescents and young adults," *Journal of Human Nutrition and Dietetics* 25, no. 1 (February 2012): 69–74. doi.org/10.1111/j.1365-277X.2011.01166.x.

114. Igor Bendik et al., "Vitamin D: a critical and essential micronutrient for human health," *Frontiers in Physiology* 5 (July 11, 2014): 248. doi.org/10.3389/fphys.2014.00248.

115. Neil Bernard Boyle, Clare Lawton, and Louise Dye, "The effects of magnesium supplementation on subjective anxiety and stress—a systematic review," *Nutrients* 9, no. 5 (May 2017): 429. doi.org/10.3390/nu9050429.

116. G. K. Schwalfenberg and S. J. Genius, "The Importance of Magnesium in Clinical Healthcare," *Scientifica* (2017). doi.org/10.1155/2017/4179326.

117. Flávia G. Cândido et al., "Addition of pooled pumpkin seed to mixed meals reduced postprandial glycemia: a randomized placebo-controlled clinical trial," *Nutrition Research* 56 (August 2018): 90–97. doi.org/10.1016/j.nutres.2018.04.015.

118. Zhaoping Shelly Li et al., "Hass avocado modulates postprandial inflam-matory responses to a hamburger meal in healthy volunteers," *Food and Function* 4, no. 3 (February 26, 2013): 384–391. doi.org/10.1039/c2fo30226h.

119. Priyanga Ranasinghe et al., "Medicinal properties of 'true' cinnamon (*Cinnamomom zeylanicum*): a systematic review," *BMC Complementary and Alternative Medicine* 13 (2013). doi.org/10.1186/1472-6882-13-275.

120. R. W. Allen et al., "Cinnamon use in type 2 diabetes: an updated systematic review and meta-analysis," *Annals of Family Medicine* 11, no. 5 (September–October 2013): 452–459. doi.org/10.1370/afm.1517.

121. N. Kizilaslan and N. Z. Erdem, "The effect of different amounts of cinnamon consumption on blood glucose in healthy adult individuals," *International Journal of Food Science* (March 4, 2019). doi.org/10.1155/2019/4138534.

122. Ahmed Salih, "Anti-diabetic and antioxidant effect of cinnamon in poorly controlled type-2 diabetic Iraqi patients: A randomized, placebo-controlled clinical trial," *Journal of Intercultural Ethnopharmacology* 5, no. 2 (February 21, 2016): 103–113. doi.org/10.5455/jice.20160217044511.

123. A. L. Francis and R. C. Beemer, "How does yoga reduce stress? Embodied cognition and emotion highlight the influence of the musculoskeletal system," *Complementary Therapies in Medicine* 43 (April 2019): 170–175. doi.org/ 10.1016/j.ctim.2019.01.024.

124. Ed O'Brien and Robert W. Smith, "Unconventional Consumption Methods and Enjoying Things Consumed: Recapturing the 'First-Time' Experience," *Personality and Social Psychology Bulletin* 45, no. 1 (June 2018). doi.org/10.1177/0146167218779823.

125. Brian Wansink and Ellen van Kleef, "Dinner rituals that correlate with child and adult BMI," *Obesity* 22, no. 5 (October 1, 2013): E91–95. doi.org/10.1002/oby.20629.

126. Sophie Kergoat, Veronique Braesco, Britt Burton-Freeman, and Marion Hetherington, "Effects of chewing on appetite, food intake and gut hormones: a systematic review and meta-analysis," *Physiology and Behavior* 151 (July 2015): 88–96. doi.org/10.1016/j.physbeh.2015.07.017.

127. Sophie Miquel-Kergoat, Veronique Azais-Braesco, Britt Burton-Freeman, and Marion M. Hetherington, "Effects of chewing on appetite, food intake and gut hormones: A systematic review and meta-analysis," *Physiology and Behavior* 151 (November 2015): 88–96. doi.org/10.1016/j.physbeh.2015.07.017.

128. K. J. Melanson and D. L. Kresge, "Chewing gum decreases energy intake at lunch following a controlled breakfast," *Appetite* 118 (November 1, 2017): 1–7. doi.org/10.1016/j.appet.2017.

129. Akitsu Ikeda et al., "Chewing stimulation reduces appetite ratings and attentional bias toward visual food stimuli in healthy-weight individuals," *Frontiers in Psychology* (February 8, 2018). doi.org/10.3389/fpsyg.2018.00099.

130. Yong Zhu and James H. Hollis, "Increasing the Number of Chews before Swallowing Reduces Meal Size in Normal-Weight, Overweight, and

Obese Adults," *Journal of the Academy of Nutrition and Dietetics* 114, no.6 (June 2014): 926–931. doi.org/10.1016/j.jand.2013.08.020.

131. Sophie Kergoat, Veronique Braesco, Britt Burton-Freeman, and Marion Hetherington, "Effects of chewing on appetite, food intake, and gut hormones: a systematic review and meta-analysis," *Physiology and Behavior* 151 (July 2015): 88–96. doi.org/10.1016/j.physbeh.2015.07.017.

132. Eva Almiron-Roig et al., "Large portion sizes increase bite size and eating rate in overweight women," *Physiology and Behavior* 139 (February 2015): 297–302. doi.org/10.1016/j.physbeh.2014.11.041.

133. D. P. Bolhuis et al., "Consumption with large sip sizes increases food intake and leads to underestimation of the amount consumed," *PLOS One* 8, no. 1 (2013). doi.org/10.1371/journal.pone.0053288.

134. Laura L. Wilkinson et al., "Keeping pace with your eating: visual feedback affects eating rate in humans," *PLOS One* 11, no. 2 (February 1, 2016). doi.org/10.1371/journal.pone.0147603.

135. Ashley E. Mason et al., "Effects of mindfulness-based intervention on mindful eating, sweets consumption, and fasting glucose levels in obese adults: data from the SHINE randomized controlled trial," *Journal of Behavioral Medicine* 39, no. 2 (April 2016): 201–213. doi.org/10.1007/s10865 -015-9692-8.

136. M. Hetherington, B. J. Rolls, and V. J. Burley, "The time course of sensory-specific satiety," *Appetite* 12, no. 1 (February 1989): 57–68.

137. E. N. Garbinsky, C. K. Morewedge, and B. Shiv, "Interference of the end: why recency bias in memory determines when a food is consumed again," *Psychological Science* 25, no. 7 (July 2014): 1466–1474. doi.org/10.1177 /0956797614534268.

138. Lizette Borelli, "The 'Crunch Effect': Tuning In To Food Sounds May Help You Eat Less, Lose Weight," *Medical Daily* (March 16, 2016). http:// www.medicaldaily.com/tuning-food-sounds-eat-less-crunch-378166.

139. Sarah Knapton, "Eat in the dark to lose weight, say scientists," *Telegraph* (February 23, 2016). https://www.telegraph.co.uk/news/science/science -news/12170702/Eat-in-the-dark-to-lose-weight-say-scientists.html.

140. Eric Robinson et al., "Eating attentively: a systematic review and meta-analysis on the effect of food intake memory and awareness on eating," *American Journal of Clinical Nutrition* 97, no. 4 (April 2013): 728–742. doi .org/10.3945/ajcn.112.045245.

141. Reine van der Wal and Lotte F. van Dillen, "Leaving a Flat Taste in Your Mouth: Task Load Reduces Taste Perception," *Psychological Science* 24, no. 7 (May 2013): 1277–1284. doi.org/10.1177/0956797612471953.

142. Jane Ogden et al., "Distraction, the desire to eat and food intake. Towards an expanded model of mindless eating," *Appetite* 62 (December 2012): 119–126. doi.org/10.1016/j.appet.2012.11.023.

143. Eva Kemps and Marika Tiggemann, "Modality-specific imagery reduces cravings for food: An application of the elaborated intrusion theory of desire to food craving," *Journal of Experimental Psychology Applied* 13, no. 2 (July 2007): 95–104. doi.org/10.1037/1076-898X.13.2.95.

144. K. Tapper and A. Turner, "The effect of a mindfulness-based decentering strategy on chocolate craving," *Appetite* 130 (November 1, 2018): 157–162. doi.org/10.1016/j.appet.2018.08.011.

145. S. Schumacher, E. Kemps, and M. Tiggemann, "Acceptance- and imagery-based strategies can reduce chocolate cravings: A test of the elaborated-intrusion theory of desire," *Appetite* 130 (June 1, 2017): 63–70. doi.org/10.1016/j.appet.2017.02.012.

146. S. Schumacher, E. Kemps, and M. Tiggemann, "The food craving experience: Thoughts, images and resistance as predictors of craving intensity and consumption," *Appetite* 133 (February 1, 2019): 387–392. doi.org/10.1016/j.appet.2018.11.018.

147. Shou Zhou, Michael A. Shapiro, and Brian Wansink, "The audience keeps eating more if a movie character keeps eating: An unconscious mechanism for media influence on eating behaviors," *Appetite* 108 (January 1, 2017): 407–415. doi.org/10.1016/j.appet.2016.10.028.

148. T. Ohkuma et al., "Association between eating rate and obesity: a systematic review and meta-analysis," *International Journal of Obesity* 39 (May 25, 2015): 1589–1596. doi.org/10.1038/ijo.2015.96.

149. Victoria Whitelock and Eric Robinson, "Remembered Meal Satisfaction, Satiety, and Later Snack Food Intake: A Laboratory Study," *Nutrients* 10, no. 12 (December 2018). doi.org/10.3390/nu10121883.

150. Brian P. Meier, Sabrina W. Noll, and Oluwatobi J. Molokwu, "The sweet life: the effect of mindful chocolate consumption on mood," *Appetite* 108 (January 1, 2017): 21–27. doi.org/10.1016/j.appet.2016.09.018.

151. Jennifer Schmidt and Alexandra Martin, " 'Smile away your cravings' — Facial feedback modulates cue-induced food cravings," *Appetite* 116 (September 2017): 536–543. doi.org/10.1016/j.appet.2017.05.037.

Index

About the Author

Susan Albers, PsyD, is a *New York Times* bestselling author and clinical psychologist at the Cleveland Clinic. She specializes in eating issues, weight management/loss, body-image concerns, and mindfulness. After obtaining a master's and a doctoral degree from the University of Denver, Dr. Albers completed an APA internship at the University of Notre Dame in South Bend, Indiana, and a postdoctoral fellowship at Stanford University in California. Dr. Albers conducts mindful eating workshops across the country and internationally.

Dr. Albers is the author of eight mindful-eating books: *Eat Q; 50 Ways to Soothe Yourself Without Food; 50 MORE Ways to Soothe Yourself Without Food; But I Deserve This Chocolate!; Eating Mindfully; Eat, Drink, & Be Mindful; Eating Mindfully for Teens;* and *Mindful Eating 101.*

Dr. Albers has been a guest on the *The Dr. Oz Show,* the *Today* show, *Access Hollywood, Hallmark's Home & Family, New Day Cleveland,* and NPR, as well as many others. Her tips, books, and programs have been featured in *O, The Oprah Magazine; Family Circle, Woman's Day, Shape, Prevention, Self, Health,* the *New York Times, Fitness Magazine, Vanity Fair, Natural Health,* and the *Wall Street Journal.* She was named a *Cooking Light* Healthy Habits Hero. Susan is a contributor to *HuffPost* and *Psychology Today.*

On a personal note, Susan is married and has two children. She loves to travel, and she enjoys food tours in every new city she visits. Her three favorite cities are New York City, Denver, and London. Her favorite go-to Hanger Management foods are salt-and-vinegar almonds and apples with almond butter. She likes collectables with green apples on them—as it is her favorite symbol and food! In her free time, Susan likes reading biographies, practicing yoga, kickboxing, and hiking. She has been to almost every national park in the United States.

Learn more at eatingmindfully.com.